Night Terrors

Troubled Sleep and the Stories We Tell About It

ALICE VERNON

ICON

This edition published in the UK and USA in 2023
by Icon Books Ltd, Omnibus Business Centre,
39–41 North Road, London N7 9DP
email: info@iconbooks.com
www.iconbooks.com

First published in the UK and USA in 2022 by Icon Books Ltd

ISBN: 978-178578-868-0
eBook: 978-178578-794-2

British Library Cataloguing in Publication Data.

A catalogue record for this book is available from the
British Library.

Typeset in Adobe Jenson by Marie Doherty

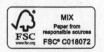

Printed and bound in Great Britain by
Clays Ltd, Elcograf S.p.A.

ABOUT THE AUTHOR

Dr Alice Vernon is Lecturer in Creative Writing at Aberystwyth University, where she teaches students the fundamentals of storytelling. Her research focuses on representations of sleep in science and culture. This is her first book.

Contents

1   Introduction   1
2   Not guilty on grounds of unconsciousness   29
3   Bedroom ghosts   61
4   Hag-ridden   89
5   Night terrors   123
6   Narrating dreams   157
7   Lucid dreaming   199

    Conclusion   227

    Acknowledgements   233
    References   235
    Notes   243
    Index   253

'Tonight, I shall strive hard to sleep naturally.'

Bram Stoker, *Dracula* (1897)

'If we pay no attention to sleep,
we thereby admit that a third of our
lives are unworthy of investigation.'

Marie de Manacéïne, *Sleep: Its Physiology,
Pathology, Hygiene, and Psychology* (1897)

Chapter 1

Introduction

In the early hours of New Year's Day, 2018, I woke up to find a stranger standing by my bed. Despite the darkness, I could see them clearly. It was a woman, and she was looking down at me. She was middle-aged, had brown, curly hair, and wore a white blouse that seemed to cast a pale glow around her.

Terrified, I sat up and shuffled away until my back hit the wall, never breaking eye contact with her for a moment. She was between me and my closed bedroom door, and I knew I wouldn't be able to get past her if I tried to run away. But as the seconds passed, my thoughts began to slow down.

This had happened before, I reminded myself. I had seen things, things that weren't really there, on and around my bed. Spiders, usually, but occasionally something bigger. People looming down at me or peering from the corner of the room. They would flash before my eyes for a brief moment and then disappear.

This woman wasn't disappearing, though.

I blinked hard, and she stayed where she was. Something was wrong. I started to panic; this wasn't like the other times,

1

with the spiders or shadowy figures. It was real. I could see the faint floral pattern on her shirt. For all that she looked harmless, like anyone you might pass on the street, I knew that she was dangerous. Behind her glare was a sinister feeling. She was going to hurt me. My heart was beating painfully fast; I wanted to run but I was trapped in the corner of my room, unable to escape. I reached across and fumbled for my bedside lamp.

Soft light melted away the dark. The woman was gone.

My shoulders dropped and I let my feet slide away from me, although I could still hear the muffled throb of my pulse in my ears. With shaking hands, I picked up the water bottle next to the lamp and took a sip.

I had gone back to my parents' house for the Christmas period, and I listened out for any sound of them stirring in the room across the hallway. My door was shut and I didn't think I cried out, but I could never be sure. I decided I wouldn't mention it in the morning.

As I started to relax, I thought about what I had seen. I tried to rationalise it and dissect it; I always feel like a bit of an idiot when I see things in the night that aren't really there, so it helps to be analytical rather than mortified. Staying up to see in the New Year, drinking alcohol late at night, the frantic piano-playing of Jools Holland as the clock neared midnight: it had all combined to make me hallucinate something far worse than normal. That was the explanation. Nevertheless, when I finally turned out the light half an hour later, I kept seeing the woman in my mind's eye. I drifted back to sleep, feeling uneasy. Haunted. I hoped I wouldn't see her again.

☆ ☆ ☆

Falling asleep is often easy for me. I have nights when it's difficult to switch off, when I've got something important to do in the morning or I'm still churning over the events of a chaotic day, but I rarely suffer with prolonged periods of sleeplessness. I wish this was as miraculous as it sounds, but it isn't. I don't sleep soundly; I sleep strangely.

Ever since I was a child, my nights have been populated by monsters, aliens, and the shadow of another me who acted without my knowledge. When I was young, I used to sleepwalk around the house or refuse to go to bed at all for fear of the nightmares that tormented me. Then, as a teenager, my sleep suddenly descended into a much more peculiar realm. Since then, I regularly wake up in the middle of the night in pure terror, having experienced a ghostly assault.

Nightmares, night terrors, lucid dreams, sleep paralysis, somnambulism and hypnopompic hallucinations are some of the phenomena known as 'parasomnias'. Even the name evokes images of ghosts and monsters, crumbling towers and overgrown graveyards. These strange states of sleep have a profound and timeless effect on our imagination, shaping art, literature and scientific investigations, and provoking paranoia of witches and, more recently, extra-terrestrial encounters. Parasomnias, even in their most bizarre and frightening forms, are more common than we might think. Recent surveys estimate that around 70% of the population will experience a parasomnia at least once in their life, with the most common forms being sleeptalking and nightmares.[1,2] The problem, however, is that a combination of not remembering what we've done in our sleep, and fearing the stigma of admitting to hallucinations, violent behaviour or erotic dreams may mean that survey results are much lower than the real prevalence. When I talk to others about my sleep, I find that sometimes people will confess that they've experienced something similar – they just didn't know it was 'a thing'. In this book, we will investigate tales of sleep disorders through history, not only to see parasomnias mythologised and fictionalised, but in order to help us to talk and to listen to stories about our own troubled sleep.

☆ ☆ ☆

I've always had the propensity to experience parasomnias, but it was only when I was a teenager that they took on new forms and a new significance. Since then, the occasional sleepwalk or bad dream has developed into something a lot more sinister.

When I was fifteen, a new teacher started at my secondary school. She was young – fresh out of university – and full of enthusiasm and bright ideas. But she took an immediate, unhealthy interest in me that slowly festered into something manipulative and claustrophobic. And now she haunts my sleep.

I only knew her for three years, but it took me a lot longer to shake off the anxiety and mistrust her behaviour caused. It was nothing scandalous or explicit, but it has done lasting damage. As far as I know, she was never questioned by other staff in the school. I don't blame any of the other adults around me at the time; in the beginning, even I didn't think things were problematic. But I suppose it was that sheltered naivety that made me a prime target in the first place. Nevertheless, I eventually began a slow and painful process of recovery. And while, mostly, I don't think about her at all during the day, in my sleep she continues to terrify me. She is the unseen figure chasing me in dreams, the shadow that floats in the corner of my room, and the vivid, firm hand that grasps my neck when I'm paralysed. In this book I call her Meredith, after *mara* – the old term for sleep paralysis. It seems fitting.

It was my last year at that school, after which I went elsewhere to do my A-Levels. At that age, I was getting restless – I wanted to move on to bigger challenges. There were some subjects that I found particularly frustrating; English was one of them. I knew that there was so much to read and learn, but we were spending term after term picking apart the adjectives and nouns in a fake county-council planning application. Some teachers took pity, slipping me old copies of *The Guardian* or recommending books and films. When Meredith arrived and quickly started doing the same, I didn't think anything of it. But I now see the difference: the culture section of a crumpled newspaper had no strings attached, but Meredith's offerings were a tangled web of secret messages and the promise of a long, uncomfortable conversation after school.

I unfortunately had English as my last lesson twice a week, and she knew that I had a ten-minute window before the bus left without me. Once I missed the bus, I'd have to wait an hour for my parents to finish work and come to collect me. Maybe it was a coincidence, but fairly early in the term she rearranged the tables and assigned me the furthest seat from the exit. With me at the back of the queue to leave the room, she could lean across the blue door frame or stop me while she slowly rummaged in her Cath Kidston bag for a new book or film that was 'a bit mature, but I think you can handle it'. From over her shoulder, I'd watch the corridor beyond bustle with pupils, then eerily empty out. I was alone with her, again.

She laid bare her insecurities in that classroom, then told me how terrible the world was in an attempt to make me feel the same way. Everyone in the staff room judged her, she said. Her friends always betrayed her in the end. She often mentioned that she 'did these things' because I reminded her of herself. 'It's scary, sometimes,' she told me. Scary for whom? I liked books, that was all, but I liked lots of other things that she didn't: astronomy, chess, *X-Men* comics, angry-girl bands. I don't think we were very similar at all, but she had a set fantasy in her mind which she projected onto me. When she found differences between us, she'd do something about it. For example, I had a long fringe that I'd do up in a quiff made rock-solid with hairspray – my friends and I had a game to see how many pencils I could hold in it. One day she came in with the same hairstyle, so I stopped doing it. Science made her nervous, she said; she pretended to throw up if I talked about a meteor shower or a newly discovered dinosaur, so I stopped talking about it. She often told me her life was overwhelming; she seemed glad when I started to feel overwhelmed myself. She wrote down a local therapist's number and gave it to me – now we *were* the same.

What I remember most about Meredith is the feeling of being smothered. Physically, she would stand incredibly close to me, but I felt emotionally trapped too. She made it clear to me – her teenage pupil she had known for a month – that she was vulnerable, and any distress, any betrayal, would seriously hurt her. When I have sleep paralysis, I feel an extreme version of this claustrophobia; I'm crushed under the intense stare of Meredith, under her hands and her sharp nails, under the weight of her own emotional problems that I don't want to exacerbate.

I become a timid teenager again, pinned through my stomach like a little beetle to a display board, unable to escape.

Most of my strange nights involve the memory of her in some way, which makes me think that my sleep disorders are a direct result of this time in my life. But, as I'll show in the following chapters, it's a little more complicated than that. It's not just for anonymity that I refer to her as Meredith; what I'm left with now is something that is quite different to who she really is. I've come to realise, as an adult and a teacher myself, that she was clearly in mental distress. It doesn't excuse how she treated me, but I think I do feel some sort of pity. However, what terrorises my sleep is nothing short of monstrous. It's a vicious cycle: every time I see Meredith, either in my dreams or as a hallucination, she becomes more frightening. The memory of that will then produce something worse, and so on. Although she represents my anxiety in a general way – if I'm worried about work, deadlines or family matters, I'll have a nightmare about Meredith – at their root, the nightmares are still also about her. It doesn't matter how my parasomnias twist her, a handful of incidents laid the foundations for years of troubled sleep.

The memory of the first time I saw Meredith appears in my nightmares quite often. It was the first day of term, and I was walking across a courtyard to get to a lesson. On the other side was a teacher, a young woman I hadn't seen before. I glanced at her out of harmless curiosity, as dozens of pupils must have already done, but the look she gave me was deliberate, intense, almost rehearsed. And I remember thinking: 'Who is that, and why is she staring at me?'

Just for a moment, I was unsettled. In hindsight, so much of the chaos that would follow was foreshadowed in those few seconds before I walked past her. Our initial encounter felt significant when it happened, but looking back adds an almost melodramatic weight to it. This is the image that repeats most often in my sleep: Meredith, standing still, silently looking at me. What she says in those looks can change – sometimes her eyes seem to plead with me, other times they are charged with ferocity. Sometimes she does more than stare at me, sitting on my chest and strangling me or dragging me down my mattress by my ankles.

I'm still not sure what Meredith wanted from me. I'm not sure she really knew, either. I think she was insecure in the choices she had made and saw in me a way to vicariously relive her adolescence. Or she felt lonely, isolated and misunderstood and wanted someone else to feel the way she felt about the world. But what followed that intense encounter by the drama studio was a long period of emotional and psychological manipulation that I now re-encounter in my sleep.

☆ ☆ ☆

The history of our understanding of sleep disorders is fascinating and twisting, advancing in some areas and retreating into fear and confusion in others. Dreams are perhaps the most interrogated, interpreted and misunderstood phenomena of sleep. For over a thousand years, they have been fictionalised, dissected, glorified and demonised in an endless cycle of romanticism and rational analysis.

It's often thought that our understanding of dreams and sleep-related phenomena moved in a uniform manner from divine inspiration or Satanic influence in the medieval era to a wholly neurological process in the present day, but it's much more complicated than that. Even today, with our knowledge of sleep stages, rapid eye movement (REM) and brain waves, there are people who consider their dreams to be of cosmic origin, or their sleep paralysis episodes as visitations from angels or aliens.

Even in antiquity, when the gods of Greek and Roman religion were a fundamental part of everyday life, stories about dreams and sleep were varied. Macrobius, a fifth-century Roman philosopher, broke sleep into five categories: prophetic vision (*visio*), nightmare (*insomnium*), ghostly apparition (*phantasma*), enigmatic dream (*somnium*), and the oracular dream (*oraculum*).[3] There is particular emphasis here on the dream as a portent.

It isn't true to say that *everyone* believed that dreams were a gift from the gods, but there were numerous ideas regarding a relationship between dreams and divine influence. In ancient Greece, for example, the god of medicine, Asclepius, was believed to have a keen interest in dreams. The process known as 'incubation' in this era involved a sick or injured person visiting a shrine to Asclepius and sleeping there. During the night, Asclepius was supposed to either cure the person's ailment or show them a dream which instructed them on the best cure or treatment.[4] The 'epiphany' dream was rather commonly reported at this time, too. Epiphanies were dreams that were thought to be a visitation from a god, but this could be very widely interpreted – sometimes the gods didn't actually appear as themselves, but their presence would be known by the message they gave. The philosopher Pliny, for example, wrote that when a man was afflicted by rabies, a god told his mother the cure in a dream. The authenticity of these dreams was said to be shown through an 'apport', some sort of physical object or sign such as a letter that symbolised the visiting god and would be left behind in the sleeper's bed. The tale of Bellerophon is a classic example. Bellerophon, a hero of Greek mythology famous for slaying the monstrous Chimera, slept at the temple of Athena in order to receive her wisdom. In his dream, Athena presented him with a golden bridle, which remained next to him when he woke up.

The vast majority of epiphanies recorded were experienced by those in positions of power – important figures whom the gods would feasibly pick out to relay a message. The messages themselves ranged from the epic to the rather trivial: from advising strategies in an upcoming war and warning of another's betrayal, to requesting that a statue of them be moved from one location to another. On many occasions, it is likely that members of the ruling class professed to receiving an epiphany dream to justify any drastic or strange decisions or to explain victories in battle – the gods were on their side and wanted them to win.

In Reginald Scot's 1584 treatise, *The Discoverie of Witchcraft*, he describes the phenomenon of sleep paralysis in a wholly corporeal, rather than supernatural, manner. He calls it a 'bodilie disease' which extends 'unto the trouble of the mind' – not a symptom of a witch's curse.[5] Scot was somewhat correct, although his explanation uses the theory of 'humours' – substances which were produced by the body and caused certain symptoms and conditions if they were deemed to be 'imbalanced'. Nevertheless, over one hundred years later, numerous people were killed as witches in Salem, Massachusetts; some of the damning testimonies that describe the victims as witches involve accounts of what sounds very much like sleep paralysis.

Sleep has always been associated with the bodily condition and the supernatural, the physical and the divine. Our understanding of sleep and its phenomena has been, and continues to be, tangled with these two threads. I want to know what's happening in my brain and my body when I lucid dream or endure sleep paralysis. But at the same time, for me, sleep is like a return to the imaginative suspicion of childhood and the fear of encounters with strange ghosts and monsters. Even now, when we know so much about the sleeping brain, all the data and explanations can't numb the absolute horror of feeling a phantom hand gripping your ankle.

☆ ☆ ☆

I was afraid of the dark as a child, brought on by an early instance of weird sleep. I was a fairly robust kid, always curious and building things and trying to make people laugh, and I was only really afraid of spiders. Dinosaurs were my absolute favourite thing (they still are), and I used to spend hours poring over gruesome illustrations in my dinosaur books. I had a very special holographic keyring which showed a velociraptor, muzzle dripping with blood, that plunged in and out of its prey's carcass when I tilted my hand. But then I started to have bad dreams, and they made me rather fearful and timid, dreading when night would arrive.

A few instances stand out in my memory, but the first was a series of recurring dreams featuring a tin man. I grew up fairly close to a small and very pretty Welsh town called Llangollen, which used to have a *Doctor Who* museum. My parents, who grew up watching the show, would sometimes take us there. The earliest memories I have of that place are ones of confusion, dark rooms and flashing lights, strange voices coming out of tall, sinister robots. I don't think I quite understood what *Doctor Who* was, so this wasn't the nicest experience. But what I remember most is the occasion when a man dressed up as a Cyberman was walking up and down the river path by the museum. I find this hilarious now, but at the time I was less thrilled to be placed in the Cyberman's arms by my enthusiastic, science-fiction-loving parents.

Then came the tin man dreams. In these, I was always being pursued by a cold, tall robot and I could never get away fast enough. Sometimes I would be in our local town with Mum, outside Woolworths, and she would be swept away in a crowd of people. I'd lose my grip on her hand, and then I would find that my legs wouldn't work; I was trying to run, but I couldn't.

The worst thing about these dreams was the noise the tin man made. It wasn't so much his actual appearance that scared me, but the heavy *whum-whum* of his metal boots coming closer and closer. He'd nearly be upon me, and then I would wake up, but for some horrible reason I could still hear the dull thud of his footsteps. I'd press my face into my pillow, clutch Doggy (a pink cuddly dog I quite literally loved to death – by the time I gave him up he was a rather macabre, one-eyed head with the back seam of his body hanging like a spinal cord) and listen as the footsteps seemed to retreat into the distance.

I now understand that this was my own heartbeat, pumping frantically in fear of the nightmare and calming down in the minutes after I woke up. I think I tried to explain this noise to my parents, but at that age I was unable to describe it in a way that made sense. To me, it was real – I was really hearing the tin man leaving my bedroom after tormenting me.

My final tin man dream took place in the playground of my primary school. The yard circled the school, and I spent many a breaktime running around it in games of tag and hide-and-seek. In this dream, I was doing just that, but with pure terror in place of fun. Wherever I ran, whichever favourite hiding spot I retreated to, the tin man soon followed me.

I clambered up the steps near the back door, wondering if I could somehow scale the wall and run home. But the tin man was suddenly there, in front of me now instead of behind me. This was it; he was finally going to get me.

He stopped. We looked at each other.

Slowly, his hands moved up towards his head. He lifted off his helmet. Underneath was a middle-aged man's face, brown hair thinning back from his temples. I had never seen him before, but I knew that this was the man who had always been under the metal suit. He didn't say anything, he didn't even change his neutral facial expression, but somehow my fear vanished.

I woke up, and I never dreamed about the tin man again.

☆ ☆ ☆

When we talk about a dream, we repackage it into a form that makes for a good story – we trim it down, remove any extraneous detail, embellish the moments of tension. The same applies to our episodes of sleepwalking or sleeptalking, or how witnesses report our strange behaviour back to us. This book, then, investigates how the darker parts of our sleep have gripped our imaginations across time and culture. From the dreams of antiquity to twenty-first-century experiments into the brainwaves of a sleepwalking human, we have sought to represent the elusive and subjective experiences of sleep in art, writing, and charted graphs.

Our dreams can tell us things about ourselves, especially if we're stressed or anxious about something. But sleep takes on a new significance in fiction; it becomes its own setting, a plot device with a plethora of uses. To show us how an upsetting event has affected the heroine in a film, we'll see her bolt up, gasping, in bed (I only occasionally do this, and I doubt it makes me look as attractively troubled as in the movies). If a character is guilty of something, they might sleepwalk or unknowingly natter incriminating information. On the other hand, troubled sleep might be presented as supernatural; ghosts and goblins haunt bedrooms, and vampires paralyse their victims during their nightly attack. But, as we'll see, these works of pure imagination aren't always easily distinguishable from real anecdotes; both share a sense of blurring between what is real and what is perceived. Throughout this book, we will examine the various ways parasomnias have been depicted: in fiction from prose to video games, in court papers, private diaries, sensational news articles, experiments, and in personal accounts shared with friends, doctors, and psychiatrists. We'll discover how sleep and dreams have been described, misrepresented, even hidden away as shameful secrets, and we'll think about how we might be encouraged to tell our own stories of troubled sleep.

☆ ☆ ☆

Bram Stoker's *Dracula* (1897) demonstrates a spectrum of representations of disordered sleep in fiction, so it's a good place to start our investigation. It has stuck with me since I read it as a teenager, but it was only while I was researching insomnia and sleep in fiction for my PhD that I realised why I liked it so much.

Dracula isn't just an infamous vampire: he is every parasomnia combined in the figure of a folkloric monster.

The book begins with the journal of Jonathan Harker, a solicitor on a business trip to Romania. His client is Count Dracula, and he stays as a guest at the mysterious man's castle while he helps to arrange the purchase of a house in London. Soon, however, he learns that Dracula is a blood-sucking monster and, while the Count prepares himself for a journey of his own, manages to escape despite his weak and terrified condition.

Among its many readings, *Dracula* can be interpreted as a novel about the anxiety of intrusions. This is quite literal when Dracula crashes onto the shore of Whitby in the ill-fated *Demeter*, immediately making his uncanny appearance known in the form of a strange, large dog leaping from the wreckage. Soon, though, he begins to invade the sleep of guests holidaying at a nearby home – particularly two young women, Mina Murray (Jonathan's fiancée) and Lucy Westenra.

As the book progresses, Mina becomes increasingly obsessed with sleep. She writes about the arrival and quality of sleep in many of her journal entries. It is sparked from observing her friend, Lucy, sleepwalking along Whitby's cliffs. From this point in the text, Mina is consumed by her preoccupation with documenting her own sleep and the sleep of others. She is agitated and restless, worried about Lucy and the still-absent Jonathan. Sometimes Mina's sleep comes easily and is dreamless, but more often it eludes her. Lucy, meanwhile, suddenly sickens with a mysterious illness. Their friend, Dr John Seward, enlists the help of his teacher, Abraham Van Helsing, to try to uncover the cause of her rapidly declining health. After Lucy's death from unexplained blood loss, Van Helsing proves that a vampire moves among them, and has added Lucy to his ranks. She is swiftly dispatched, and the rest of the group, now including Jonathan, set their sights on Dracula. This is where the book seems to become particularly preoccupied with sleep. For Mina, Lucy's night-time walk is understood to be the pivotal moment when her friend crossed a threshold into Dracula's realm. As with sleepers through the ages, Mina experiences the vulnerability of unconsciousness – that her sleep might also be intruded upon by the monsters of folklore.

When Mina then begins to be visited by Dracula, she exhibits signs of nearly every parasomniac condition. The first example appears to be a kind of sleep paralysis, in which Mina is overcome by a 'leaden lethargy' that 'seemed to chain [her] limbs'.[6] Following the episode, she writes that she will 'strive hard to sleep naturally', illustrating her need for healthy sleep and identifying the episode as akin to Lucy's somnambulism. After she is attacked by the Count, her sleep is documented by others. In Jonathan Harker's journal a few nights later, he describes being woken up by Mina 'who was sitting up with a startled look on her face', and she exclaims that there is someone in the corridor. Upon being told that there is no one there but Quincey Morris on guard duty, Mina sighs and easily slips back into sleep. This half-awake, hallucinatory conviction of a dreadful presence bears all the traits of night terrors. The following morning, Mina demands to be hypnotised by Dr Van Helsing. The description of this scene seems to parallel hypnotism with troubled sleep; during the session, she mimics the childlike obedience observed during Lucy's episode of sleepwalking, and when she awakens from her trance-like state she asks, 'Have I been talking in my sleep?' As we'll see in Chapter 2, a form of hypnotism in the Victorian era was often aligned with sleepwalking, and Stoker seems to be demonstrating this idea here.

Mina's symptoms of parasomnia seem to worsen in stages. Through sleep paralysis, she loses control of her limbs; through night terrors she appears to hallucinate frightening images; and finally, under hypnosis, she loses all autonomy and falls into the same state of somnambulism as Lucy.

Sleep is a transitional space between wakefulness and an unconscious abyss, between life and death. Parasomnias, particularly when episodes are not remembered, can be a liminal state in which the body moves and exhibits personality and emotion, but the waking, rational self is effectively 'dead'. Vampirism in *Dracula*, then, is a physical existence between life and death and between wakefulness and sleep. Dracula has now become a stereotypical figure of the undead, but for Mina he is a symbol of trauma and of guilt. In the book he is a kind of synecdoche for troubled and unnatural sleep. Moreover, she considers sleep as an external force that *comes* to her – in much the same way as she is visited by the Count – rather than recognising it as a bodily function originating within herself.

The very idea for *Dracula* is said to have come to Stoker in a nightmare. When I read it now, it is less about Dracula's blood lust and desire to colonise the world with the undead, and more about a kind of contagious parasomnia. Nightmares lead to lucid dreams, from which hypnopompic hallucinations, sleep paralysis and somnambulism might develop.

Ghost stories, particularly during the nineteenth-century boom in the genre, feature plenty of incidents that blur the line between sleep and the otherworldly. They often focus on the bedroom as the scene of a haunting, and it's usually an unfamiliar setting for the protagonist – a hotel, or as a guest in a creepy mansion. Again and again, these stories feature spooky manifestations witnessed by protagonists on the edge of sleep. In Edward Bulwer Lytton's 'The Haunted and the Haunters' (1859), the narrator wakes to 'two eyes looking down at me from [a] height' and finds himself 'weighed down by an irresistible force'.[7] This is what we now know as sleep paralysis, a sense of immense pressure often accompanied by a frightening hallucination of a malevolent figure.

The terrifying climax from M.R. James's ghost story 'Oh, Whistle, and I'll Come to You, My Lad' (1904) presents a bed as the site of abject horror. The protagonist, Parkins, is on a holiday, and while walking along a beach he finds a whistle half-buried in the sand dune. Naturally, he blows it. Later, back in his twin room at the hotel, something odd begins to happen to the spare bed: it looks as though it has been slept in. The following night, the true haunting occurs. Parkins wakes in the night to find the sheet in the other bed moving, then rising, and assuming the outline of a figure. In the moonlight, Parkins sees that the sheet has 'a horrible, an intensely horrible, face of *crumpled linen*'.[8] A literal ghost in a bedsheet. As with many of these stories, the protagonist is introduced to us as a staunch sceptic of all things supernatural, but his experiences convince him of an afterlife. This is the hold strange sleep has over us: it can make us believe in ghosts, even though the only ghosts we see are the ones we create.

Beds are places of rest, safety, security, but only if your sleep is peaceful. For insomniacs, the bed is a cruel tormentor; for those of us with parasomnias, the bed is a haunted crypt.

✮ ✮ ✮

When I was a PhD student, I experienced sleep paralysis for the first time. It brought the memory of Meredith back in a way that gave me terrible anxiety for a few months. In fact, for a while, it felt as though I had gone right back to being fifteen again. I couldn't think about anything else but Meredith, such was the horrifying clarity with which she had reappeared in my sleep. About halfway through my thesis, I realised that my interest in sleep wasn't so much about insomnia, which I've never really had, but in the weird dreams and hallucinations that I've experienced all my life. I think I had always wanted to write about sleep, but when I was drawing up my PhD proposal, I wasn't quite ready to look so closely at my own situation. Towards the end, it was all I wanted to do. And so I started to think about this book.

While we'll be looking at modern diagnoses and treatments, this book won't offer suggestions of cures for these sleep disorders. Instead, it is primarily interested in examining the effect of parasomnias on society and how these phenomena have been interpreted and misinterpreted in the past. From witches to aliens to sleepwalking murderers, we will explore how representations of sleep disorders have developed, and how we learned to separate sleep from the supernatural. By examining these stories, and looking inwards to our own experiences, perhaps we'll get to know our sleep better.

The book's journey begins with the first parasomnia I ever experienced: sleepwalking. Also known as somnambulism, it is a common parasomnia, and can range from the sleeper making small movements to committing elaborate crimes. This opening chapter will look at some of the curious examples of sleepwalking in history and culture, from young women whose nightly walks became a source of entertainment, to people who committed murder in their sleep.

I then move to a darker part of my sleep. One of the first ways Meredith irreversibly changed my sleep was in the form of hallucinations, when I started seeing spiders in my bed. When I opened my eyes, one would be scuttling next to my pillow, or aiming for my forehead as it descended from the ceiling. After a brief moment of panic, I would realise that I had been hallucinating. These dream-like images onto the waking mind are known as hypnopompic hallucinations, and they're vivid enough to be easily mistaken for something real. Chapter 3 will discuss examples of hypnopompic hallucinations, focusing particularly on their influence on Victorian ghost stories.

I often see things that aren't really there, but sometimes I *feel* them, too. I wake up with my body heavy and rigid, and a sense that something, someone, has their hands around my neck or is dragging me down my mattress by my ankles. Sleep paralysis was once interpreted as being 'ridden' by the incubus or succubus, a shadowy, impish figure that sought to squeeze the life out of its helpless victim. It led to suspicions of witchcraft, demonic possession, and ghostly visitations. In the next chapter, we will look at the history of our interpretations of sleep paralysis, and the ways in which its control over our bodies and minds has emerged in fiction and art.

Night terrors, on the other hand, often lack the lucidity and sense of being awake that are characteristic of hypnopompic hallucinations and sleep paralysis. Known as *pavor nocturnus*, this parasomnia is frequently seen in children, but can also affect adults. The sleeper is suddenly seized by a fear so strong that they often scream or hurt themselves and others in a frantic attempt to flee the object of their distress. Chapter 5 explores the scientific and cultural depictions of the condition, and brings it to life through the experiences of sufferers like my cousin.

Chapter 6 will explore our unrelenting fascination with dreams and nightmares. Sigmund Freud emphasised our need to understand this nightly phenomenon in *The Interpretation of Dreams* (1901), but many earlier, and now largely forgotten, texts provided the foundations for his theories. This chapter will celebrate some of the pre-Freudian pioneers of dream research, looking at how their ideas predicted some of our most recent sleep discoveries. As well as providing endless scientific and psychological mysteries, dreams can also be a valuable source of creativity. Robert Louis Stevenson, for example, relied on his dream adventures to provide inspiration for his stories.

I have always been a vivid dreamer. Dreams are colourful, tactile, immersive dramas that cling to me like a dazzling cape for the duration of my day. If the dream was happy or exciting, I can feel it warming my general mood. If the dream was distressing, it becomes an almost physical weight on my shoulders, and if I was hurt in any way I can often sense a dull prickling at the location of the dream-injury. My childhood nightmares terrified me beyond any other experience in my life, to the point where I couldn't sleep in my own bedroom. For me, dreams aren't just the debris of a good night's sleep. They deeply affect me. I write them down, analyse them like a painting or a poem, chew them over at the back of my mind. If my dreams suddenly became shallow and dull, I would feel as though I had lost an important piece of myself. Good or bad, they are still an essential part of my life.

But when I was entangled with Meredith as a teenager, my dreams opened up like an old gate in an overgrown garden.

Over and over again, I dreamt of the corridor leading up to her blue door, and of being in her classroom. Then, one night, I realised the truth of the situation: I wasn't cringing under Meredith's intense stare, but asleep in my bed. I became awake within a dream. This phenomenon, known as lucid dreaming, has been written about for centuries but because it is a rare and fantastical experience, until recently it was kept on the fringes of sleep research. It has been discussed with scepticism; prior to modern experiments proving its occurrence, the only evidence for lucid dreaming was the personal testimony of those who had experienced it. The work of Stephen LaBerge in the 1980s, its representation in films such as Satoshi Kon's *Paprika* (2006) and Christopher Nolan's *Inception* (2010), and recent successes in inducing the state, have contributed to its prevalence in modern psychology. Chapter 7 will explore the wonderful and bizarre phenomenon of lucid dreaming, revealing historical examples and modern research, as well as discussing how it can be used for therapeutic and creative purposes.

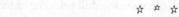

Night-time, for me, is a source of both fear and familiarity. I used to dread its arrival when I was a young child; the way the house seemed to hold its breath and bedrooms became menacing, shadowy spaces. It felt oppressive, as though I was being watched by monsters I couldn't see myself. As I got older, my relationship with the night changed, and I discovered that it could be soothing as often as it was scary. It stopped being a writhing, shapeless terror and became something warm and familiar like a big, brave dog curling itself around me.

It's for this reason that, at least at this point in my life, I yearn for the dark evenings of autumn and winter. I like some aspects of summer; the flowers, the interesting bugs, the way a cold beer becomes extra satisfying. But the hot, inescapable sunshine and the starless, navy-blue nights of west-coast Wales make me feel as though I'm in a place where I don't really belong, like a tropical fish in an aquarium.

Just before the coronavirus lockdown in early 2020, I went to the Science Museum in London for the first time. I think my inner child resurfaced that day, and I remembered how cool science – especially space – could be. And in the long, troubled summer that followed, the memory of this trip was one of the things that sustained me when I felt particularly low. In the autumn, as the nights started to get longer and darker, I bought myself a pair of astronomy binoculars. This might sound a bit sad, but the first time I took them outside and looked up, I nearly started crying.

Throughout the winter, I went out to look at the stars whenever the sky was clear enough. I would wrap up warmly, fumbling in my thick gloves, and step outside onto the dark little terrace with my comically giant binoculars. With the lenses pressed up into my eyes, it felt like I was somewhere else. I was in this safe, enclosed, quiet little world with Jupiter and Saturn and the Pleiades. I could hear the waves sloshing against the promenade in the distance, the sound of seagulls and other animals nestling down, and those cosy clangs of pots and pans as people made dinner in the houses behind me.

This is how I like my nights to play out. After a little while stargazing, I go back up to my flat. I switch on the small, warm lights and lamps I have dotted around, and I make a cup of camomile tea. I started drinking this when I was younger, on holiday and so desperately bored in my hotel room that I sampled all the teas in the caddy just for something to do. Camomile tea smells like the sweepings from a hamster's cage, but somehow I acquired a taste for it and now I drink it almost every evening. I'm also a big fan of classic Hollywood movies – the more melodramatic and fabulously costumed the better – so I might watch something before heading to bed. Then I usually read a few pages from a non-fiction book. Lastly, I do a bit of meditation. Nothing fancy, and only for a few minutes; it's just a way of calming down my breath and my muscles if I've gone to bed feeling tense about something. It helps me let go of the day.

And then, I melt into bed, into the darkness.

I have a habit from my childhood of imagining some sort of story as I drift off; they used to be stories in which I was a glamorous hero with every single superpower combined, but in adulthood it's become more of a boring visualisation exercise. I fantasise about planting seeds in a garden, or wandering alone around the Natural History Museum, or revisiting scenes in a film I recently watched to try to figure out what on earth was going on. After a few minutes of this, my thoughts become syrupy-slow. I try to focus on the image of my hands tying string around a tomato seedling, but then I forget what I was doing, what I was thinking about just a second ago.

It may or may not be related to my parasomnia bingo card, but sometimes I experience an odd sensation just before I fall asleep. It is so subjective, possibly more so than my other sleep phenomena, that it's quite difficult to describe. I have a sense of where 'I' am in my body – I'm the twittering little voice behind my eyes, floating in some abstract space in my skull. But I know *where* that is, like being able to navigate the living room in thick darkness – you know where you are in relation to the rest of the room and furniture. When this sensation happens, I have the most peculiar distortion of my position in the world. It feels as though 'I' have shrunk inside my body; I'm no longer in a living room but in a vast football stadium that keeps growing and growing. My eyelids feel as though they're miles away. Sometimes it affects different parts of my body or the space I can sense around me – my head might suddenly feel massive, or the bed shrinks to the size of a box of matches. It stops as soon as I open my eyes.

I used to have this a lot as a child, and it would frighten me quite badly – now I only tend to feel like this if I've gone to bed immediately after returning from a party. It's not even the alcohol that does it; just the buzz and energy of a social gathering seems to set this off, as though my brain is rebelling from the sleep I'm trying to force it to have. For a long time, I thought this happened to everyone until I wrote a scene about it in my PhD novel, showed it to a friend, and quickly learned otherwise. It seems similar to a condition called, ironically, Alice in Wonderland Syndrome. The sensation of growing and shrinking is compared to Alice in Lewis Carroll's classic children's story, when she becomes large or tiny depending on what she eats and drinks. It's harmless, as far as I can tell, and I actually find it quite entertaining to feel my head become cavernous (which might be caused by the alcohol). But I wonder if it is part of whatever makes me experience strange things in my sleep. It is, after all, a type of hallucination, a strange distortion of reality.

Despite my troubled sleep, I feel the most like myself at night. In the daytime, I feel tense, rushed, constantly trying to do something or be somewhere or feel as though I'm making good use of my time. Summer is the same; I find it inescapable and suffocating, and I yearn for the cold and the dark. The night – proper, pitch-black night – is different; I relax, I slow down and become more curious and attentive to the world around me. At night, in a dark room, I can plunge into a film, the television screen flickering light across the room. I can be cosy, quiet, alone, and I can go out with my binoculars to see the stars and planets so far away from me. And then I can sleep, and dream, and experience a deeper, stranger part of myself.

I love sleep, even though sleep doesn't always love me back. The things I see at night scare me, but they also fascinate and sometimes excite me. They are as much a part of me as my small stature or mousy hair or love of dinosaurs. But I've pushed these odd sleep experiences to the back of my mind for a long time, and I want to shine a bit of light on the darker part of my life. By researching these parasomnias, talking about them, reading anecdotes from people who've experienced the same thing, I want to understand them, and myself, better.

Some of my favourite times of the academic year are our Open Days when we welcome prospective students and their parents and generally eat a lot of cake. We usually hold a 'meet the department' event, where we do a quick introduction to our work and maybe read or talk about some of our recent research. Over the last few years, I've been talking about this book and reading some draft material. Without fail, a handful of people come up to me afterwards with a mixture of horror and delight on their faces, eager to tell me about their own weird sleep experiences that, until now, they didn't realise had a name. And sometimes, there's even a sense of relief; they may never have told anyone else about the monkey they hallucinated on the curtain pole one night, but suddenly they want to tell me.

This is also why I wanted to write this book. I want more conversations with people about their nightmares, their lucid dreams, their sleepwalking antics. They are far more common than we realise but, as we'll see, their historic connection to demons and the supernatural continues to have a lingering effect. Even modern discussions of parasomnias are riddled with misunderstandings and superstitions, but we shouldn't be afraid to talk about them. I want us to talk about these phantoms of sleep with the same frequency and cultural acceptance as our conversations about insomnia. By paying attention to my own sleep demons, I'm hoping that you might be able to do the same.

☆　☆　☆

It's time for bed. My bedside lamp is dim, and my bed is warm and soft. I've spent some time reading a non-fiction book, but now the words seem to be blurring into each other and I find my eyes scanning the same sentence without taking in its meaning. I close the book, and put it beside me. I turn off the light; my room becomes dark. The headlights of an occasional passing car slice across the curtain pole.

I grab a fistful of duvet, close my eyes, and roll onto my right side. I think about an infinite row of plant pots and a bottomless packet of sunflower seeds, and I imagine puncturing the cool, damp soil with my finger and dropping a seed into the hole. I suddenly think about a scene from *The Exorcist*. I try not to think about *The Exorcist*. Back to the sunflower seeds.

One by one, I watch them grow before me; I see the yellow of
their petals, yellow, the yellow submarine bath toy I had as a
child, warm water, warmth.

I fall asleep.

Chapter 2

Not guilty on grounds
of unconsciousness

'What if I wake up somewhere else?'

It's an intrusive thought, like a dog barking at a visitor at the door, that often comes when I'm on the edge of sleep. My eyes snap open and I stare into the darkness of my bedroom. I then spend a few nervous minutes picturing myself, bare feet and baggy pyjamas, suddenly regaining consciousness on Aberystwyth's promenade. Carefully, I go over my plan. I would go to the 24-hour shop on Terrace Road. I would explain myself as calmly and lucidly as possible, and hope that the staff could sort me out. I keep my keys on my bedside table, in the hope that even in my sleep I would remember to take them with me. It would never happen anyway, I tell myself as I roll over and close my eyes again.

But still, I occasionally find myself out of my bed, getting ready to walk up to campus at three o'clock in the morning. Recently, I began to help an invisible friend who had lost something in my kitchen; I woke up with my hand on the light switch and midway through proclaiming that I'd find it.

I seem to be able to catch the tail-end of these episodes – there's a moment where my sleeping and waking selves merge. I slowly become aware that my determination to do something – to prepare a lecture, put my shoes on to go grocery shopping, make a cup of tea for a phantom visitor – is ludicrous. It's like working on a jigsaw; I realise, piece by piece, that I'm in my pyjamas, that it's the middle of the night, that the semester is over, that I'm by myself. Sheepishly, I form the full picture. I've been sleepwalking.

☆　☆　☆

Also known as somnambulism, sleepwalking is the phenomenon of moving and undertaking complex physical actions despite being asleep. These actions can range from walking across the bedroom and back to cooking a three-course meal or even driving a car. It's a fairly common parasomnia in children, but can persist into or even develop in adulthood. Usually, the sleepwalker's eyes are open – but with a far-away stare that can be quite disconcerting. To wake a sleepwalker during an episode can disorient or frighten them, and so it's best to talk to the person calmly and try to guide them back to bed. Most often the episode passes without incident, but there have been famous cases in the past of violence, accidental self-harm, and even murder committed during sleep.

A report published in 1869 by the *Chicago Medical Journal* described a strange case of somnambulism. Written by Professor J. Adams Allen, it relates the nightly exploits of an unnamed friend – one of his own medical students.[1] The young man had a history of sleepwalking, which seemed to have begun in 1847, after the student sustained a head injury from falling down a set of stairs that had no rail to hold on to. While sharing accommodation, Adams Allen witnessed him getting dressed and wandering around before getting back into bed. Every time Adams Allen told him about what had happened in the night, the student couldn't remember doing any of it.

Shortly after his somnambulism began, the student inherited an antique – and dreadfully out of tune – bass violin. Adams Allen describes his student as a musical man, and fondly recalls the way the student became determined to tame the awkward notes of the instrument. In fact, he was so determined that his sleepwalks took him back to the room where he kept the violin, and he would continue to play it with even more concentration than he showed during the day.

What I admire most about the way Adams Allen begins this story is the warmth in his description. He obviously cared about the student, and writes about the sleepwalking incidents with a mixture of amusement, curiosity, and concern. I'm sure most of us would be annoyed to hear an out-of-tune violin strike up at two o'clock in the morning, but Adams Allen calls the experience 'wonderful'.

But the student's somnambulism nearly caused him to give up his blossoming career in medicine. In the early 1860s, in the depths of winter, he was responsible for the care of a very poorly man. He visited the patient in the early evening, and said he would come back as soon as he could the following day with a change of medication if the man didn't seem to be improving.

As promised, the next morning he saddled his horse and went to see his patient. Remarkably, the man seemed a great deal better. The student asked how and when it had happened, and was horrified at the man's answer.

'Immediately after taking the powders which you had given in the night,' said his patient.

The student, as he found out from the patient's family, had arrived between two and three o'clock in the morning. There was nothing about his behaviour, besides the strange time of his visit, that struck the family as odd. His conversation with them continued where he had left it earlier that evening; he stopped the medication he had previously given the patient, and instead had him take the first dose of the new powders he was going to bring on his next visit.

Fortunately, the sleepwalking student brought the medication he would otherwise have delivered in the morning. But his horror seems to scream out through Adams Allen's writing; what if he had brought something poisonous, instead? What if he had returned, as promised, in the morning, and found his patient dead because the family trusted him too much to question an out-of-character visit? How could he possibly stop it from happening again? It's easy to see why the student nearly left the profession. Somnambulism can make you afraid of yourself.

☆ ☆ ☆

In my parents' house, the house I grew up in, there is still a baby-gate at the top of the stairs. The wood is chipped here and there, and the little knob to control the latch is loose and squeaky with age. But, by force of habit, it is clicked shut every night, even when I'm not there.

The baby-gate is a reminder of that strange part of myself who came out in force when I was a child. The 'other' me who, at breakfast, Mum would say she had encountered on the landing. Mum is a light sleeper, and will often wake up if she hears movement in the house, so she would hear me come out of my bedroom. She had learnt how to deal with me when I was sleepwalking; she would talk quietly, try to learn what sort of situation I thought I was in, and play along with the narrative in such a way that I could be persuaded to get back into bed.

As far as I know, the worst thing I've ever done is rip a page out of a book. I was eleven years old, and I woke up one morning to find a scrunched-up ball of paper on my carpet. Confused, I smoothed it out and was horrified to discover that it was from the book I was currently borrowing from one of my sisters. I didn't tell her, and I never gave the book back. I still feel bad about it.

But where my book-destroying antics are harmless, the serious crimes committed by sleepwalkers have fascinated scientists and the public for centuries. How do you prosecute a person who was unconscious during their moment of violence? How do you, the person on trial, defend yourself for something you don't know you did? Could you ever come to terms with that unknown criminal inside yourself? It's a thought that horrifies me. At night, when I'm nervously visualising my pyjama-clad walk through town, there's a much deeper worry of what else I could do. To sleepwalk is to live with a part of yourself you can't ever know, whom you have to trust will stay in bed and not go on an uncharacteristic rampage in the middle of the night.

33

As with all books and articles on parasomnias, I'm drawn to reading about the crimes committed by sleepwalkers. I can't help myself. Maybe I read about it so that the sleepwalking part of myself will take note of the consequences – a kind of warning to that strange 'other' me. I can spend hours trawling through Old Bailey sessions papers, looking for cases of somnambulists on trial for a crime they simultaneously did and didn't commit.

☆ ☆ ☆

On 26 May 1853, a street in Hyde Park was shaken by the actions of a supposed sleepwalker.[2] At seven o'clock in the morning, thirteen-year-old Frederick Smith woke up to find the family servant holding a carving knife to his neck. Sarah Minchin, four years his senior, knelt on his arms and pressed the blade into his skin.

Frederick cried out: 'Oh, Sarah! Sarah!'

Sarah covered his mouth, and said nothing.

Also resident in the house was Charles Cushen, who worked in Frederick's father's grocery shop. Cushen heard the boy's frightened cries and ran into Frederick's bedroom. The scene was bloody; Frederick, defending his already wounded neck, had caught the knife in his hands. Cushen took the knife away without meeting resistance, and Sarah seemed to collapse in an insensible heap. Still, she had made no sound. Moreover, she was dressed only in her nightgown, 'as if she had just got out of bed'.

Sarah was carried, eyes closed and apparently unconscious, out of the house by a police officer. She finally woke up on the cab journey to the station.

During the trial, there was discussion of somnambulism. Cushen remained convinced that it was all an act on Sarah's part; she had really intended to kill Frederick. The question of sleepwalking was posed to a house surgeon at St Mary's hospital, who seemed not to believe in somnambulism at all and dismissed the claim. Sarah's mother was called up to provide evidence, and spoke of how her daughter had bad dreams and 'screams out a good deal in her sleep,' for which reason they slept in the same room together. I think of the baby-gate at my parents' house.

Sarah, it was revealed, had been in employment in two different places prior to the Smiths' house – each for a year at a time – and had worked for the Smiths for around three months. This rapid change of employment, of different beds in different environments, wasn't picked up by the jury. And, in the end, she was convicted of unlawfully wounding and confined for three months.

This case is one of several that contributed to a developing discussion on the idea of a 'second self'. Philosophers, physicians and early psychologists were beginning to investigate the biological causes of sudden mood swings, epileptic fits or changes in energy from wakefulness to stupor, and aspects of insanity. The idea of the 'other' self emerged, of multiple identities within a person, and questions were asked about whether everyone had a part of themselves they couldn't control – and if they couldn't control it, were they then relieved of responsibility for the other's actions? Furthermore, if *everyone* had this propensity, then the emergence of this unconscious self couldn't be associated with other known forms of insanity. It was a time of real moral and mental dilemma, especially in a culture where propriety and reservation of character were incredibly important, and the idea that everyone had a part of themselves who could commit terrible violence was difficult to digest. But it did lead to changes in the courtroom, and around twenty years after Sarah Minchin's case, the verdict of 'not guilty on the grounds of unconsciousness' was recorded for the first time.

The case occurred in 1876, when Elizabeth Carr stood trial for cutting her four-month-old baby's hand off with a table knife, subsequently killing the child.[3] While not a case of sleepwalking as such, the accused's actions are similar to the unaware and automatic actions of a somnambulist. Her statement before the Magistrate reads: 'I hope you will not think I was in a clear state of consciousness when I did it.' The witnesses and a doctor all attested to Carr's history of similar 'fits', in which she suddenly slumped and then proceeded to wander around like a sleepwalker, with no idea or memory of what she had done.

Dr Edward Merrion took to the stand, both to give his medical opinion and to provide evidence of his previous encounters with Carr. He was a physician at the Hospital for Diseases of the Nervous System, and had been a practitioner for forty years. He told the court that Carr had been his patient since 1871, and had 'not a doubt but that she was absolutely unconscious of what she was doing'. Regarding the case, Dr Merrion explained that Carr thought she was preparing a slice of bread and butter, and mistook her baby's hand for the loaf. He argued that what Carr suffered from was not in any way linked to insanity, and that her actions were akin to the twitching or continued movements of a centipede after its head has been cut off. The evidence from several people of Carr's history of episodes, combined with the discussions prevalent at this time, led to the verdict of 'not guilty on grounds of unconsciousness'.

There have been several more recent cases of sleepwalking crimes. In 2009, Brian Thomas from south Wales, supposedly gripped by a nightmare, strangled his wife to death while they slept in a campervan on holiday. As with Sarah Minchin's case 150 years earlier, the court heard of Thomas's history with sleep disorders – particularly night terrors. At the end of the trial, he was cleared of murder on the grounds that he had not been able to control his body's actions.[4] Similarly, in North Carolina in 2015, Joseph Mitchell was found not guilty after smothering his young son while sleepwalking.[5] Even the charge of manslaughter was found to be inappropriate in a case where the defendant was unconscious at the time of the murder. The news reports of these cases make for uneasy reading; there is a sense of abject horror common to all of them, and it's demonstrated most strongly in the sleepwalker. I find my breath gets shallow when I try to imagine what it must be like to wake up to wreckage that you unknowingly caused. And even though the jury might be sympathetic, how would you ever make peace with that side of yourself that had the ability to kill someone?

I have eventful nights several times a week, and while the hallucinations and nightmares are enough to spook me for a few hours, my potential to sleepwalk is what causes me the greatest concern. At the end of this research, if I manage to feel a little less afraid of what I might experience in my sleep, I know that my dread of somnambulism can't truly be defeated. Then again, perhaps that's what keeps my sleepwalking self in check.

Sleepovers were an issue for me as a child. It wasn't so much that I was afraid of what I'd do in my sleep, but I was nervous that my friends would see me do it. There is nothing crueller than a group of ten-year-old girls. I thought that if they saw me sleepwalk, they'd make sure it haunted me for the rest of my days.

As an adult, romantic relationships dwindle very quickly for me. For the most part, I'm just too comfortable in my own company. I'm like a cat, demanding attention for a little while and then scampering off. It's only when I'm a few months into dating someone that I realise I'm much happier by myself. But I'd be lying if I said my sleep didn't factor into my preference to be unattached. I think it's because I'm protective of my sleep. Actually, it's more like I'm protective *of myself* when I'm sleeping. I want to keep my sleeping self away from observation. Whenever I'm dating someone, I'll leave their house or kick them out of mine when I want to go to sleep. If I try to stay the night, I just won't sleep at all. Maybe, one day, I'll be able to trust that part of me with another person. At the moment, though, my nights are still unpredictable and my parasomnias are fluctuating and morphing all the time. I don't think I can bear the mocking 'guess what you did last night' from a partner just yet.

☆ ☆ ☆

In the nineteenth century, the act of observing the exploits of young female sleepwalkers became a popular subject for scientific treatises. Adapted from a lecture given at the Springfield Lyceum in Massachusetts in 1834, L.W. Belden's *An Account of Jane C. Rider, the Springfield Somnambulist* is a detailed description of a seventeen-year-old girl's experiences with sleepwalking.[6] Or rather, it's about how her sleepwalking was witnessed by medical men.

She's described at first as having 'plump and rosy cheeks', indicating that her healthy appearance is somehow at odds with her somnambulism. Belden, the family doctor, explains that he was called one night to attend Jane. She was out of bed and delirious, mistaking Belden for her father and leading him to think she was deranged.

Over the next few pages, Belden describes her condition as becoming more severe. She got up and set the table perfectly for breakfast – a task she performed every morning – and was then angry when she later awoke and saw that someone had apparently stolen her job. On another occasion, and for reasons Belden doesn't really explain, Jane seized a knife that was being used to fasten shut the door at the top of the stairs. She sleepwalked into the room where Belden and a few others were sitting, furiously threw the knife at their feet, and exclaimed, 'Why do you wish to fasten me in?'

This part of Belden's book reminds me of sharing a room in a holiday cottage with one of my sisters. I was twelve or thirteen years old. The room was next to the kitchen, and our parents were sleeping in the other side of the house.

'I'm not happy,' my sister said. 'I don't like that it's next to the kitchen.'

'Why?'

'You're going to sleepwalk and get a knife.'

'No, I'm not,' I said, as indignantly as I could.

But I did get up in the night. Perhaps my sister's suspicion, even fear, of me planted the sleepwalking seed in my brain out of spite. Fortunately, I didn't pick up a knife from the kitchen. I walked over to the chest of drawers, picked up her little tube of tea-tree moisturiser, and quietly set it down on the table between our beds. My sister watched me in terror as I wandered around the dark bedroom.

Observation plays a key role in Belden's book. The appendix of *An Account of Jane C. Rider* features 'Letters from several gentlemen' testifying to having witnessed Jane in her home during a 'paroxysm' of sleepwalking. A few of these letters thank Belden for inviting them to watch Jane while she slept.

These gatherings involved more than simply watching Jane, however. Belden goes into detail about a number of experiments performed while Jane was sleepwalking. These mostly involved Jane's sight; Belden would blindfold her with silk handkerchiefs and then persuade her to navigate a room, sew, or read books and notes she had never seen before. Allegedly, she would act as clearly and as lucidly as though she were awake and her eyes were open.

The spectacle of the somnambulist was simultaneously reflected in the popular psychical research movement of the nineteenth century. A sudden fascination with trance states – heralded by German physician Franz Friedrich Anton Mesmer, who came up with the idea of 'animal magnetism' to hypnotise and control another human being – and female mediums performing for audiences led to sleepwalking becoming entangled with the paranormal. The term 'somnambulism' was forced to split into 'natural' and 'artificial' forms. Artificial somnambulism was the name given to the hypnotised state popularised by public séances. In these events, a female medium and male mesmerist would take to the stage; the man would make 'magnetic passes' over the woman, using the energy in his hands to divert and manipulate the energy in her body. Then, when magnetised and induced into a somnambulistic state, the medium would be open to communicate with the spirit world. It was a hugely fashionable form of entertainment at the time, with notable fans including Charles Dickens and Sir Arthur Conan Doyle.

With interest in somnambulism becoming tied to belief in the supernatural, it's no wonder that fiction became rife with sensational and portentous sleepwalkers. In fact, the tormented soul possessed in sleep by their own guilt became quite the trope. Said to be the first detective novel, Wilkie Collins' *The Moonstone* (1868) features a priceless diamond that goes missing shortly after it is given to a young woman for her birthday. Its disappearance is seemingly inexplicable, with red herrings leading to dead ends and false accusations. Towards the end of the novel, Mr Franklin Blake, who was responsible for the safekeeping of the diamond before it was presented, discovers that he had unconsciously taken the Moonstone and lost it to thieving hands. He had been wracked with nerves about keeping the diamond secure, and this mental state had moved him to want to find a better place to hide it. In order to find out where and how he inadvertently 'stole' the diamond, several characters recreate the conditions of the fateful night and observe Blake repeat his unconscious walk through the house. While his trance-like state is caused by ingesting opium, rather than 'natural' somnambulism, Blake's horror at not knowing his own movements at night is very much in line with court records and news reports of criminal sleepwalkers.

It seems as though Wilkie Collins was fascinated by these sensational articles. They do make for good stories, after all. Later in his life, he returned to this trope in his short work of fiction from 1881, 'Mr Policeman and the Cook', also known as 'Who Killed Zebedee?' Try not to picture the lolloping abdomen-on-a-spring from *The Magic Roundabout*. This story is very close to some of the sleepwalking crimes that were reported and exaggerated for public consumption, more so than in *The Moonstone*. The story is narrated by a man on his death-bed, recounting an unsolved murder that occurred during his time working for London's police force.

One night, a woman runs into the station declaring that there has been a murder at the boarding house where she is employed as a cook. A young woman has killed her husband, Mr Zebedee, but she did it in her sleep.

The narrator and the station's Inspector rush to the scene of the crime, where a doctor gives the diagnosis: Mr Zebedee has a knife plunged in his back, and is very much dead. They first question the landlady, Mrs Crosscapel. Her statement of the events reads rather like a dramatic extract from a court case:

> 'Soon after three this morning,' says she, 'I was woke by the screams of Mrs Zebedee. I found her out here on the landing, and Mr Deluc, in great alarm, trying to quiet her. Sleeping in the next room, he had only to open his door, when her screams woke him. "My dear John's murdered! I am the miserable wretch – I did it in my sleep!" She repeated those frantic words over and over again, until she dropped in a swoon. Mr Deluc and I carried her back to the bedroom. We both thought the poor creature had been driven distracted by some dreadful dream. But when we got to the bedside – don't ask me what we saw; the Doctor has told you about it already. I was once a nurse in a hospital, and accustomed, as such, to horrid sights. It turned me cold and giddy, notwithstanding.'[7]

The narrator finds Mrs Zebedee crouched on the floor in the corner of the bedroom, with her dead husband lying in a pool of blood on the bed beside her. Again, we get the link between the somnambulist and the ghost or possessed person when Collins writes: 'She stared straight at us without appearing to see us. [...] She might have been dead – like her husband – except that she perpetually picked at her fingers, and shuddered every now and again as though she was cold.' On the floor next to the bed, they discover a book that the wife had been reading: *The World of Sleep*.

Mrs Zebedee recovers enough to tell her story. Prior to her marriage, she had worked as a servant in Dorset. In that house, it was a rule that she couldn't sleep alone because of her 'occasional infirmity of sleepwalking' – one of the other female servants had to sleep with her, with the door locked and the key hidden under a pillow.

On the night of her husband's murder, they were sitting in bed together. Mr Zebedee had found *The World of Sleep* at a railway book stall and decided his wife would very definitely like to read it before going to sleep. Mrs Zebedee reads aloud to him from this book until he falls asleep, and then she continues to read to herself. She soon reaches a chapter 'which took hold on my mind', describing an anecdote about a man who stabbed his wife to death while sleepwalking.

Mrs Zebedee finds herself both horrified and fascinated by the book, and reads late into the night until she falls asleep. But she wakes suddenly, and discovers her husband's body next to her.

The rest of Collins' story is a bit strange and loses some of the intrigue and tension that it started with – perhaps this is why it has fallen into obscurity in comparison to his other works. The knife used to kill Mr Zebedee becomes the main clue; Mrs Zebedee has never seen it before, and it is mysteriously engraved 'To John Zebedee, from —'. The police, taking Mrs Zebedee's word that she has never seen the knife before, very quickly acquit the wife of murder and we never hear from her again. When the narrator does discover the real murderer, he feels too sorry for the person to do anything about it, and this is what he confesses on his deathbed. Mrs Zebedee, who was so fraught with guilt and had entirely convinced herself that she was the murderer, that this ghostly, unknown part of herself had killed the man she loved, disappears from the story. Her tale feels rather unresolved, and she didn't exactly get justice for the attempt to frame her for her husband's murder.

But perhaps that's part of the point. The sleepwalkers in treatises, newspapers and other anecdotes from this period all seem to share a common trope of exploitation. The sleepwalker is exploited for a sensational newspaper story, or put on display for a room of medical men and made to do tricks and experiments while they are completely unaware. The same is true for Mrs Zebedee; the sleepwalking side of herself is exploited by the murderer in an attempt to get away with the crime.

Another good example of a literary sleepwalker is seen in Thomas Hardy's 1891 novel *Tess of the D'Urbervilles*. The novel follows an ill-fated young girl, Tess, whose unfortunate encounter with a minor aristocrat leads to a string of terrible choices that culminate in murder. Halfway through the book, Hardy includes a scene in which the sensitive Angel Clare, Tess's husband, sleepwalks into the room where Tess is in bed. Hardy writes:

Not long after one o 'clock there was a slight creak in the darkened farm-house once the mansion of the D'Urbervilles. Tess, who used the upper chamber, heard it and awoke. It had come from the corner step of the staircase, which, as usual, was loosely nailed. She saw the door of her bedroom open, and the figure of her husband crossed the stream of moonlight with a curiously careful tread. He was in his shirt and trousers only, and her first flush of joy died when she perceived that his eyes were fixed in an unnatural state of vacancy. When he reached the middle of the room he stood still and murmured, in tones of indescribable sadness—

'Dead! Dead! Dead!'[8]

He lifts Tess in his arms and carries her out of the house. Tess stays silent, observing Clare with a mixture of curiosity and fear. Clare takes her to a graveyard, where he places her down in an empty stone coffin. As seen in the case of Sarah Minchin, he suddenly falls down in a deep slumber. He does not wake up; but is able to move, still in a somnambulic state, when Tess gently encourages him to walk back to the house.

Before they had gone to bed that night, Tess had revealed her dark history with Alec D'Urberville. Caused by his 'mental distress', Clare's sleepwalking seems to be animated by the emotions he suppressed during their waking conversation. Angel's loss of bodily control reveals another side to his character, and presents a rather sad image that the relationship with Tess is at its closest when Angel is unconscious.

☆ ☆ ☆

In 1830, a young Scottish physician and writer called Robert Macnish published *The Philosophy of Sleep* – an extensive analysis of disorders and phenomena. As he notes in the preface to the second edition, 'So far as I know, this is the only treatise in which an attempt is made to give a complete account of sleep.' He endeavours to describe the spectrum of sleep disorders and sleep-like states, from dreams to drowsiness, providing plenty of case studies from his own practice of medicine. While some of Macnish's theories on sleep have been proven inaccurate, he is still influential in the history of our understanding of sleep, and some of the texts we'll encounter in later chapters reference or pay homage to his book. With each edition Macnish added new findings and ideas, but his examination of sleep was cut short by a fatal typhus fever in 1837, when he was 34 years old.

In regards to sleepwalking, Macnish describes it as a direct result of dreams. When a dream is 'of so forcible a nature as to stimulate into action the muscular system,' he says, somnambulism occurs. In other words, he believed that sleepwalking happens when a person acts out their dream.

He was partly correct, but we now know of the existence of REM behaviour disorder (RBD). It was first described in humans in 1986 by a team of sleep researchers led by Carlos Schenck, who were investigating the 'aggressive behaviours during sleep' of four men aged 67–72 years old.[9] This parasomnia occurs when the paralysis that stops you from acting out your dreams doesn't work. If you dream about making a cake, you'll start cracking open invisible eggs. More troublingly, if you sleep next to a partner and dream of getting into a fight, the partner may suffer the blows. Moreover, exhibiting signs of RBD can be an early indication of a degenerative disease such as dementia or Parkinson's. We'll revisit RBD later in the book, as it also has connections with night terrors.

In sleepwalking, however, there is no particular known cause or trigger. It could be genetic, it could be down to excessive tiredness, or even changes in hormones. And unlike RBD, there isn't evidence of a dream or conscious thought behind the sleeper's actions. The sleepwalker may, in the morning, remember some part of what they were doing, or they may find a witness's description of events familiar, as if recalling a dream. In 2000, a group of Swiss neurologists led by Claudio Bassetti discovered that the part of the brain that handles our intentions when we're awake remains dormant during episodes of sleepwalking.[10] Whatever a somnambulist does, it comes from somewhere separate to their waking self – a mixture of movements formed by memories, patterns, and reflexes.

☆ ☆ ☆

The stories of my own episodes of sleepwalking come from other people, told to me over breakfast the next morning. Mostly, it was my Mum who discovered me scurrying into my parents' bedroom or hiding Doggy in the airing cupboard, and she would give me a comedic retelling of her encounter with my other self. My favourite story happened when I was around thirteen years old, and I still laugh when I think about it now.

As I've mentioned, my Mum is a light sleeper, and that night she heard me get up and walk across the landing. She listened out, ready to come and find me if I wasn't well in the bathroom. But there was no sound of the bathroom floor creaking under my feet. Puzzled, she got out of bed to see what I was doing.

I was standing perfectly still near the stairs. I had the strange, glazed expression Mum recognised as a sign I wasn't truly awake. Even stranger, though, was the way my hands were out in front of me, palm-up and pressed together as though I was cradling something very fragile and important.

'Alice? What are you doing?' she whispered.

I looked up at her. 'Mum, I have to give this cake to Gwen Stefani.'

When Mum told me about it in the morning, her impression of my matter-of-fact tone of voice had me nearly crying with laughter. It was clearly a very important errand and I couldn't afford to waste time chatting.

Remembering the usual routine, Mum said, 'Well, it's the middle of the night. Can't you give it to her in the morning?'

I considered it for a moment. I nodded. A perfectly reasonable request. Gwen could wait. I got back into bed, and when I woke up in the morning I had no idea that I had been sleepwalking.

☆ ☆ ☆

The nightly exploits of the young Victorian somnambulist Jane C. Rider were just a small part of a larger cultural phenomenon. The figure of the pretty female sleepwalker, with her vacant, otherworldly stare and billowing white nightdress, drifted through the Victorian imagination in fiction and in true (or mostly true) anecdotes. During the wave of fascination with the occult, young women and girls were often paraded as the medium through which the spirit world communicated; sleepwalkers, then, were perhaps of particular interest because they juxtaposed the dread of the afterlife with the allure of vulnerable femininity.

Sensational newspapers such as the *Illustrated Police News*, for instance, often featured articles about the dangerous wanderings of sleepwalkers. A good example is from the American version of the *Illustrated Police News*, dated 1877, with the headline: 'A Pretty Somnambulist'.[11] In St Louis, twelve-year-old Laura Speer was observed sleepwalking by her guardians, Mr and Mrs Prior. Laura appeared at first in the Priors' bedroom, and then retreated into the corridor. The Priors followed, and watched with horror as she approached the rickety ladder to the skylight. She began to climb, and quickly opened the hatch that led onto the roof. This was apparently too much for Mrs Prior, who had to retreat back to bed. Mr Prior continued to follow, and ascended the ladder to watch Laura. The article states that she 'began to walk back and forth, perfectly silent, with her arms hanging listlessly by her side, and her head inclined forward, as if she was looking immediately in front of her feet.' She was close to the edge of the roof, and to fall would be a twenty-metre drop to certain death.

After a few minutes, Laura stopped pacing and went back to the skylight. Mr Prior ducked out of the way to let her pass. She took no notice of him, and calmly descended the ladder and tucked herself back into bed. Other than being a little cold from the night air, Mr Prior found her to be completely healthy.

While the article is entertaining in its emphatic description of Laura's dangerous situation, the final paragraph is particularly interesting. The following morning, Mrs Prior told a neighbour about Laura's antics. The neighbour related a local rumour – a lady had seen 'a white object on the roof of the Prior house at a late hour of the night, and that she believed it was a ghost indulging in a moonlight ramble on the roof.' Clearly, the night

Mr and Mrs Prior followed Laura was not the first occasion on which she had sleepwalked out of the skylight. The accompanying illustration to the story shows Laura in a ghostly appearance; she stands on the edge of the roof, her hair is loose and billowing behind her, and her white dress glows against the dark shading of the night sky. Ironically, the image above Laura is for a similarly sensational story about a 'suicidal phantom' leaping off a cliff. Their pictures seem to complement each other, and it further provokes the association of sleepwalkers with the supernatural.

The illustration of Laura is preceded in culture by numerous other depictions of the spectral somnambulist. One of the most striking is John Everett Millais' painting 'The Somnambulist' (1871). It shows a woman, only a little older than Laura, walking barefoot along the edge of a coastal path. Her hair is darker than the night sky around her, and her white nightdress laps at the ground like sea foam. There are lights far in the distance; presumably the house from which she has wandered. Hanging limply from her right hand is an unlit chamberstick – eerily showing that she is not using it to see her way. Nevertheless, her eyes are wide open and peering fixedly at something in front of her. It is, put simply, quite a creepy painting.

Sleepwalking wasn't only a Victorian fascination, even if there are plenty of examples of its hold on the public imagination. A notable depiction can be found in William Shakespeare's violent tragedy, *Macbeth*, believed to have been first performed in 1606. Macbeth, a Scottish general, is given a message by three witches that he will become King of Scotland. His wife, Lady Macbeth, is a woman of ruthless ambition, and she encourages him to murder the current ruler, King Duncan. However, their actions are met with suspicion, and Macbeth and his wife commit further murders to ensure the safety of their rule over Scotland. Macbeth's fellow general, Banquo, who accompanied Macbeth in hearing the witches' prophecy, is particularly sceptical of Duncan's sudden demise. Macbeth hires assassins to see that Banquo is swiftly silenced.

Sleep is mentioned throughout the play as a kind of judgemental, malevolent force. In particular, it is the *lack* of sleep that troubles Macbeth as guilt and paranoia of discovery consume him. After the murder of King Duncan, Macbeth claims to hear a voice cry, 'Macbeth does murder sleep.'[12] For Macbeth, it is insomnia through which his remorse manifests itself. It's a little different for Lady Macbeth.

Following Banquo's murder, we get a curious, and somewhat notorious, scene of Lady Macbeth sleepwalking. Act 5 begins with a Doctor and Waiting-Gentlewoman discussing Lady Macbeth's nocturnal wanderings. The Doctor is sceptical, but the Gentlewoman insists that she has witnessed these events herself:

Since his majesty went into the field I have
seen her rise from her bed, throw her nightgown upon
her,
unlock her closet, take forth paper, fold it, write upon't,
read
it, afterwards seal it, and again return to bed, yet all
this while
in a most fast sleep.

It is night, and the Doctor and Gentlewoman are holding vigil to see if they can catch Lady Macbeth in the act. Sure enough, she enters the scene holding a thin candle and speaking in strange, disjointed sentences. This is where we get some of *Macbeth's* most memorable dialogue:

> Out, damned spot; out, I say. One, two,— why,
> then 'tis time to do't. Hell is murky. Fie, my lord, fie!
>   a soldier
> and afeard? What need we fear who knows it, when
>   none can
> call our power to account? Yet who would have
>   thought the
> old man to have had so much blood in him?

Lady Macbeth wrings her hands during this scene, scrubbing away blood that only she can see. Guilt troubles and transforms her sleep; her act of sleepwalking breaks down her cold, ruthless demeanour to reveal the madness beneath. For the watching Doctor, it allows him to piece together some of the 'foul whisp'rings' he has heard. Through witnessing Lady Macbeth sleepwalk, he becomes suspicious of her part in the recent spate of murders. Her parasomnia betrays her.

Swiss painter Henry Fuseli (1741–1825) captured this moment in 'The Sleepwalking Lady Macbeth' (1784). Where Millais' painting shows an eerily calm somnambulist, Fuseli captures the violence of the parasomnia. Lady Macbeth holds a flaming candle aloft, though it looks remarkably like a dagger. But it's her eyes that draw my attention. In *The Illustrated Police News* article, Laura Speer's eyes were depicted as closed under heavy lids; the subject of Millais' painting had a relaxed, glazed expression. In Fuseli's image, her eyes are wide with terror and madness. Her head is slightly turned away, as though fighting the direction in which her legs are unconsciously taking her. She is not ghostly here, but rather possessed and demonic. At the time of *Macbeth*'s first performance, the common term for sleepwalker was the Latin *noctambulo*, or 'nightwalker'. As Elizabeth Hunter points out, this term had multiple connotations – among them, 'nightwalking' was used to describe the flight of witches.[13] To have troubled sleep in the seventeenth century, therefore, was more readily seen as an act of transgression and re-emerging guilt. The shift in depictions of the female sleepwalker, from the mad Lady Macbeth to the eerily vulnerable Laura Speer, reflects changing cultural attitudes to the supernatural. As we move away from a belief in witches and devils and into the mysterious realm of the spiritual, the sleepwalking woman shifts from sinful to ethereal.

☆ ☆ ☆

Somnambulists are often associated with possession and the supernatural; in fiction, their actions are either ghostly repetitions of past treachery as we see in *Macbeth* or, like *Tess of the D'Urbervilles*, strange glimpses into the future. They are observed, and it is the observers who gather meaning from the sleeper's movements or speech. Yet the person most unsettled by a sleepwalker is the sleepwalker themselves. Franklin's sense of self-loathing in *The Moonstone* when he learns of his opium-induced sleepwalk is palpable. Every morning is like a crime scene – sometimes quite literally. You have to piece together what you might have done based on what has changed in the environment around you. What is missing from the fridge?

How did the vase on the mantelpiece get smashed? Why is your work bag filled with teaspoons?

Shirley Jackson, a mid-twentieth-century American writer famous for her horror and thriller stories, continues to explore the relationship between sleepwalking and the supernatural beyond the Victorian era. One of her best-known texts is *The Haunting of Hill House* (1959). It follows the story of Eleanor Vance, an odd and lonely young woman desperate to flee her current living situation. An academic, Dr Montague, invites her to join him in an experiment to see how a group of people with a prior supernatural experience react to staying in a notoriously haunted house. Eleanor is scouted because of a childhood incident involving a shower of rocks that may or may not have been a result of telekinesis.

She arrives at Hill House and ghostly things immediately start to occur, but they seem to be focused *on* Eleanor, as though the ghost has picked her out from the rest of the group. Reminiscent of the Victorian tradition, Jackson draws a thin line between sleepwalking and ghostly possession. Eleanor becomes convinced that the ghost is inviting her to stay for ever, that she finally has a permanent home. It reaches a crescendo, and Eleanor seems to lose herself in a somnambulistic state.

This book is enjoyable not just because it's deliciously creepy, but also because there are passages where the strangeness of sleep is brought to the fore. There's a moment when Eleanor, sharing a room with fellow participant Theodora, thinks she is lying on the bed and holding Theodora's hand. Eleanor wakes up, but discovers Theodora on the other side of the room. But it's in the final act, when Eleanor is gambolling through Hill House in a mad daze, that the book makes us question what is really happening; is this the work of Eleanor's own mind, or has she been overwhelmed by a malevolent power? Can it be both?

In another of Jackson's works, a short story called 'The Tooth', there is a sense of trying to capture the feeling of a dreamlike state. 'The Tooth' is a dentistry nightmare made manifest, throbbing with Jackson's signature uncanny chirpiness in the face of acute psychological horror.[14] There are several layers and ways of reading this story. At its very surface, middle-class housewife Clara Spencer embarks on a solo trip to New York to have a tooth removed. Self-medicating for the pain, she is as high as a kite on codeine, sleeping pills and whisky, and the anaesthetic she receives at the dentist only further plunges her into a state of floating delirium. The story becomes very strange and hazy. Clara enters the dental surgeon's operating room as though she is in a somnambulistic state. Before she becomes unconscious under the general anaesthetic, the cheery doctor says, 'All you've got to worry about is telling us all your secrets while you're asleep.' When she wakes up, this is Clara's first concern. Not of the success of the operation or how she's feeling, but what she did in her sleep: '"Did I talk?" she asked suddenly, anxiously. "Did I say anything?"' Throughout the story, there's a sense that Clara is barely clinging on to her sense of self; with the tooth removed, she falls into a delusion in which she can't remember who she is. To read this story is to get close to the feeling of emerging from a sleepwalking episode. This is one of the things I like best about Jackson's writing, because the sensation of sleep disorders is so difficult to put into words and yet she captures it with spooky accuracy.

Jackson's work was inspired by her own history of parasomnias. She was particularly prone to sleepwalking, and had a lifelong interest in dreams, visions and delusions that appealed to her preoccupation with the supernatural. In one of her lectures, 'How I Write', she relates an anecdote about the writing process of *The Haunting of Hill House*:

> Two weeks ago, I had written part of the beginning of the book and was having a great deal of trouble making it go together and could not find a suitable name for my secondary female character. One evening, I had been at it for a couple of hours, typing and growling and throwing pages on the floor, and finally I decided to give up. I told my husband that I was going to have to put the book aside, maybe even start another book, maybe never go back to this one again, and I stomped furiously up to bed.
>
> The next morning, when I went to my desk, I found a sheet of typing paper; it had been taken from the pile at one side of the desk and set right in the middle. On the paper was written, 'oh no oh no Shirley not dead Theodora Theodora.' It was written in my own handwriting, but as though it had been written in the dark.
>
> I have always walked in my sleep, but I don't think I have ever been so frightened. I began to think that maybe I had better get to work writing this book awake, because otherwise I was going to find myself writing it in my sleep, and I got out the typewriter and went to work as though something were chasing me, which I kind of think something was. Since then, the book has been going along nicely, thank you, and my female character Theodora is turning out quite well.[15]

It's unclear how much of this actually happened; as we often see in this book, stories of troubled sleep are repackaged and embellished to make them more entertaining. But I definitely think there is truth in it; a large part of the experience of sleepwalking is to find messages, though not necessarily literal, written messages, the morning after. And that can be quite scary and sinister, as Jackson describes. You have no idea what you might be capable of, which is one of the biggest anxieties slowly festering in *The Haunting of Hill House* and several other of her works.

Jackson's anecdote seems to return to the supernatural tones of sleepwalking stories from the previous century. Perhaps the 1950s rise in sleep clinics and rapid developments in neuroscience shed so much light on these darker parts of sleep that, for Jackson, the sense of mystery and dread was being lost. Against these new understandings of sleep, Jackson's work instead clings to the shadowy corners of the human mind.

Sleepwalking, then, is about a loss of control over ourselves – of coming into contact with another, possibly unpleasant self who crawls out at night. We've seen stories throughout this chapter of people being alarmed to learn that they sleepwalk, and this is what horrifies me, too.

☆　☆　☆

Self-control is quite important to me. I'm trying to be a bit better at spontaneity, but mostly I find comfort in knowing what I'm doing and where I'm going. I enjoy a drink – a cold beer with my colleagues on a summer's evening on the seafront, or a warming whisky at Christmas – but the feeling of being drunk, even just a bit tipsy, is something I really dislike. I'm quite self-conscious about the way I talk; I stumble over my words rather a lot, as though my mouth and my brain are out of sync with each other, and this makes it hard to speak up or contribute to discussion sometimes – I know I have a good idea, but if only I could just directly beam it into everyone's heads instead of having to bumble through the sentence like a toddler in a sports day sack race. I think teaching has helped, but having anything more than two drinks in an evening makes me pretty unintelligible, and that leads to a lot of internal cringing and embarrassment. This is the same feeling I get from sleepwalking; of not being in control of what I do or say, but often just catching enough of the tail-end of it to know that I did do or say something weird.

While I don't sleepwalk as much or as severely as I used to as a child, sleeptalking is something that I often find myself doing. It's never much, just a word or a phrase, but the noise of it wakes me up. If I'm staying over at my parents' house for a little while, I always tense up when I know I've been sleeptalking. I strain my ears, listening through the dark to hear any signs of my parents acknowledging that Alice is at it again.

☆　☆　☆

The stories of sleepwalking we've seen in this chapter all share a sense of unease, of the dread of secrets coming to light. Somnambulists cannot trust themselves, nor are they trusted by those who watch them. The sleepwalking woman, in particular, conjures both the horror of a duplicitous personality and the tantalising image of the ethereal feminine. The tales of pretty young girls docilely wandering to precarious places seems to have been of particular interest to Victorian readers. Their fascination with death and spiritualism perhaps fuelled this storytelling trend; the somnambulist trod the thin boundary between sleep and wakefulness, between life and death. In fiction, their condition becomes a plot device. Just as ghosts are said to repeat their movements in the space they haunt, so too do sleepwalkers take familiar routes and reveal to the observer the things they repress while awake. This is the only non-REM parasomnia that is continuously used in narratives. From the murderous sleepwalker to the voyeurism involved in documenting their actions, this parasomnia lends itself to thriller writing.

Despite their uncanny appearance, somnambulists are often used in melodramatic, but nonetheless fairly realistic, stories. But other sleep disorders – particularly those that produce hallucinations – have a much more speculative influence on the imagination. They have haunted sleepers for centuries, and given rise to countless ghost stories and anecdotes believed to be genuine supernatural encounters. In the following chapter, we will explore the parasomnia of hypnopompic hallucinations – the very vivid and often terrifying experience of encountering something in the bedroom that really shouldn't be there.

Chapter 3

Bedroom ghosts

In July 2018, a woman appeared at my bedside every night for a week. It was during a period when I was moving flats in Aberystwyth. On the first night, I saw her at the foot of my bed with a young boy at her side. They looked Victorian; the child wore a dull-brown waistcoat and the woman had on a white bonnet that was luminous in the dark. Neither figure was particularly threatening, but even so, I was terrified. In the warm night, I had tangled myself in a thin blanket, and I struggled to get free. I trembled and shuffled backwards until my back hit the hard wood of the headboard. In the next moment, both figures had gone.

She came again the following night. This time, she was alone. And for the rest of the week, I didn't see the boy again. But she seemed to become larger and stronger each time she appeared.

On the last night, I woke into a strange delusion. Again, the woman was there. She had moved, though. She wasn't at the foot of my bed; she was standing over me. Her hair was a rich colour, like red wine spilled on an oak table, but it hung long and limp as she looked down at me. I had a flood of memories that started

61

well before that week, almost as though I had known her since I moved into my studio flat three years earlier. There was a sense of history, this time, and of a relationship that was about to be torn apart. Steadily, over the week, she had noticed my books disappear, my drawers and cupboards becoming empty, my shoes vanishing from their space by the door.

She didn't want me to leave.

That thought was something solid and real – information as basic and true as my address or date of birth. We stared at each other for a few moments, and I found myself completely taken in by a delusion. I *knew* who she was. I even had memories of seeing her in the past. And I was chilled by the certainty with which I understood her reason for appearing to me every night.

I just had to get through the last night, and then I would go to my new, safe, ghost-free bedroom and I'd never have to see her again. I clung to that thought like a rope.

Then she was gone, and the memories dissolved. I felt as though I had been bewitched, and suddenly the spell had lifted and I could think clearly again. I had never been so frightened of a hallucination before, not just because it was so prolonged but because I had been briefly convinced of things that were purely in my imagination.

These visitations happen to me a few times a month. I'm fairly used to them, but never had I seen something consistently over several nights. That week was the closest I've been in my adult life to rekindling my childhood fear of the dark. It was the closest I could ever feel to being haunted.

There were several reasons why she could have shown up. I had just handed in my PhD thesis, a relief so massive that my body celebrated with an attack of shingles – a feisty revival of the chicken pox virus that should otherwise stay dormant in the body unless, of course, you do a PhD. It was on the left side of my forehead and up my scalp, and I occasionally still have a quick jab from nerve damage that feels as though someone has raked a sharp fingernail through my hair. The UK was also having the longest, weariest heatwave I had ever known, and trying to sleep at night was proving to be uncomfortable and claustrophobic.

I also needed to move out. I was being kept on as a part-time teacher in the department, but there were a few reasons why I no longer wanted to live in the flat where I had written my thesis. I had a week to move to a different place across Aberystwyth – a rather brutal task I was determined to do by myself rather than hire a van. I didn't have any furniture to shift, but it still wasn't the best idea I've ever had. Then, once the move was done and I was at my parents' house for the rest of the summer, I was due to give a speech at my sister's wedding (which, uncharacteristically, I'd left to the last minute to write). It was a particularly frantic time of blistering heat, stress and upheaval. An open invitation for hallucinations.

☆　☆　☆

There are two main forms of sleep-related hallucination: hypnagogic and hypnopompic. You may have heard of hypnagogic hallucinations, and have likely experienced them; they are the flashes of images or patterns that appear against our eyelids when we're close to falling asleep. Hypnopompic hallucinations are much rarer, and involve the projection of dream-like images, feelings or sounds onto waking perception. It often occurs in the first moments after waking up; a presence such as a person, monster, or animal will appear for a second or two – long enough for the viewer to react – before disappearing.

Before I began to research the stories of sleep disorders, I used to think that what I was experiencing was a night terror. It happened at night, and often filled me with terror. But night terrors, as I'll show you in Chapter 5, involve the sleeper being seized by overwhelming fear and often letting out a blood-curdling scream. In the morning, however, nothing of the night's drama is remembered, whereas I can always recall what I've seen or done. I am awake when I hallucinate, whereas those who suffer with night terrors are still asleep during the episode.

It was only towards the end of my PhD that I learnt about the phenomenon of hypnopompic hallucinations. I was reading Oliver Sacks' *Hallucinations* (2012), and his chapter on visions on the edge of sleep features the following explanation:

> Hypnopompic hallucinations are often seen with open eyes, in bright illumination; they are frequently projected into external space and seem to be totally solid and real. They sometimes give amusement or pleasure, but they often cause distress or even terror, for they may seem charged with intentionality and ready to attack the just-awakened hallucinator.[1]

Rather than occurring in the internal mind, then, hypnopompic hallucinations appear in the space beyond the sleeper's body. And the sleeper can react to the hallucination – by running away or trying to fight it, for example – before the image disappears. I was always awake and aware, and I would react in some fight-or-flight manner to what I saw.

My July experiences aside, what I see is never the same two nights in a row. Sometimes I will sit staring at whatever has manifested in my room, and sometimes I seem only to catch the phantom just as it disappears – as though I wasn't meant to see it at all. More often than not, I manage to reason with myself (and with the hallucination) that what I'm seeing isn't real. But occasionally, the hallucination will carry a delusion with it. I become convinced by a story, or by memories that aren't mine.

The hallucinations are usually quite random, but just like dreams they can be connected to something that happened to me during the day. After the move in 2018, for example, while I was at my parents' home, I went for a walk with Mum to a local pub. They live in a rural village, and the journey involves navigating some narrow roads with farmland on either side. Beneath the hedgerows were little stalks of bright orange berries. I hadn't seen them before, and Mum identified them as the highly poisonous cuckoo-pint. They looked like something out of a fairy tale; enticing but evil. That night, I woke up in the middle of the night to a soft glow around my bed. I sat up and saw a carpet of illuminated berries sprouting up from my mattress. These were highly fragile, and for a moment I wondered how I would get out of bed without damaging them. I knew I would have to be very careful. As I looked around me, the hallucination vanished and I was left in the dark, feeling like a bit of an idiot.

☆ ☆ ☆

When the brain is asleep, its attention is focused inwards. There is still a slight awareness of external stimuli, but otherwise the brain's functions are far fewer than during wakefulness.

Hallucinatory sleep phenomena such as hypnopompic hallucinations, however, have been linked to sudden 'micro-arousals' in the brain's activity which can bring a person out of sleep before they're ready. In other words, while your brain is in its immersive dreaming state, you suddenly wake up for a moment. Your eyes are open and your waking brain functions begin to return, but just for a few seconds the slow-wave patterns of REM sleep persist, and the vivid images associated with dreams slip into the world around you.

Hypnopompic hallucinations are still a puzzle to neuroscientists. They can affect healthy brains, but can also be present in – and be a precursor to – a number of illnesses. Among these is dementia with Lewy bodies, named after Friedrich H. Lewy who first discovered these abnormal protein deposits in the brain which cause the disease. Dementia with Lewy bodies includes the symptom of distressing hallucinations and delusions alongside the more common signs of dementia. Italian neuroscientist Pietro Tiraboschi and his team investigated an 80-year-old woman with Lewy bodies dementia in 2013.[2] She experienced hypnopompic hallucinations several years before her dementia diagnosis, but over time the hallucinations moved from being purely within the realm of sleep to occurring at random during the day.

It is also a symptom of schizophrenia. But hypnopompic hallucinations can affect people without any other neurological disorders. There must be an overlap somewhere – something that links people who experience this parasomnia despite the differences in the health of their brain. A team at the University of Western Australia have been trying to identify this relationship. Led by Flavie Waters, the investigation outlines the similarities and differences between the hypnopompic hallucinations of those with and without schizophrenia.[3] According to Waters and her team, one of the fundamental differences is how the hallucinations affect the brain afterwards. Waters uses the term 'sleep-related' to separate 'normal' (i.e., arising from a healthy brain) hypnopompic hallucinations from the hallucinations of neurological disorders. In a healthy person, the hallucination quickly fades. This is how I experience them; I'm pulled into the hallucination for no more than a few seconds, and then I realise that it was all in my half-awake mind. In a person with schizophrenia, however, the delusion associated with the hallucination persists, and may even cause a permanent change to the person's sense of self.

A study led by Felicity Waite in the University of Oxford provides a fascinating example of this difference.[4] Waite's team are trying to develop a form of Cognitive Behavioural Therapy (CBT) for treating the sleeping problems of schizophrenia patients. One of the patients in the study suffered a hypnopompic hallucination in which she could smell gunpowder. This was accompanied by the delusion that she was in a war zone – something she had never actually experienced. After the hallucination faded, the patient believed that 'her life was not her own', and that she was actually someone else who had been at war. For schizophrenia patients, therefore, these hallucinations can often displace and create new realities.

But despite these differences of experience, Waters and her team found that the common root of hypnopompic hallucinations seems to be the thalamo-cortical circuit of the brain. This part of the brain regulates sleep and produces the images of dreams, but is also involved in morbid hallucinations resulting from psychological and neurodegenerative diseases. In other words, hallucinations arise when the parts of the brain activated during REM sleep also become active during the day.

I started to hallucinate soon after I started my A-Levels at college. During that period, I had begun the painful process of trying to detach myself from Meredith. For a while, I was terrible at it; I'd manage a week or so, and then she'd send me a nice text and I'd curse myself for being a horrible person. I was having a lot of nightmares about her, though. My sleeping mind was showing me an image of her I couldn't admit to during the day. Every time I had a nightmare about her, she would become more monstrous in my mind, leading me to have worse nightmares. After a while, these dreams started to do strange things. Because of the recurring patterns, I started to be able to force myself awake. This led me to start lucid dreaming, too – the experience of knowing you're dreaming while you're dreaming that I'll discuss in Chapter 7. If I didn't like my dream, I would drag myself out of it like walking through thick mud. It seemed to flip a switch in my brain, though; around the same time as I began to lucid dream, I would sometimes wake up and hallucinate for a few seconds.

At first, I always saw spiders. I'd wake up in the middle of the night to see a spider next to my pillow or dangling by its web an inch above my face. I have a phobia of spiders, so I would scramble to get myself as far away as possible – only to find that there was nothing on or near my bed to begin with. Over the years, however, the things that appear to me have become more complex. I see figures – usually women – looming over me. No matter how demonic or completely harmless they appear, I always react with a feeling of primal terror. My heart races, and before I can think, I'm lashing out with my fists to protect myself.

While most of my memories of Meredith have dulled over time, there is still one incident that makes me wince. I think it's this moment in particular that forms the rotten root of my hypnopompic hallucinations. I had just started at a local college, and the distance away from her was finally making me realise that her behaviour towards me wasn't normal. But by that point, I was too entangled in her messy emotional blackmail. And that was why, despite now being at a different school, I ended up going back once a week with two of my fellow ex-pupils to help with an afternoon drama club.

On one of these afternoons, I found myself rumbling with animosity towards Meredith. I didn't want to be there. I didn't want to be with her.

She picked up on it instantly.

'Stay behind afterwards,' she said, looking me up and down with peculiar intensity.

I shouldn't have gone in the first place, but it would have meant giving an excuse and then dealing with a string of manipulative texts. Plus, I think I wanted her to see me in a bad mood. But as soon as she spoke to me, my resolve crumbled.

When the drama club students started putting on their coats and filing out of the door, I tried to sneak out with them.

'Miss Vernon!'

Ah.

'You're not going.'

Meekly, I stayed behind. I watched my two friends leave without me. I watched the last pupil exit, Meredith shutting the door behind him.

She walked over to where the chairs were stacked; she pulled out two and clanged them down. Then, one in each hand, she dragged the chairs across the drama studio floor.

She looked at me. 'Sit down. You're not leaving until you tell me what's wrong.'

Sitting there next to her, dodging her questions, I felt like she was ramming cotton wool down my throat. My anger was being smothered, and all the things I had worked out to say to her were now lost in suffocating fluff.

We were sitting there for a long time. I kept saying that I was fine, but she was insistent on finding out what was bothering me. She wouldn't let me out until she was satisfied.

'My A-Levels are stressing me out,' I muttered to my shoes. And then, because Meredith would always make fun of me for being interested in science, I came up with the perfect excuse. 'It's like you said; I shouldn't have taken Physics.'

Either she accepted that as truth or it really was getting late, I'll never know, but she finally let me leave. It had done irreparable damage, though. The sensation of entrapment, of vulnerability, of being at the whim of a scrutinising, possessive force, had lodged itself firmly in my brain.

My hypnopompic hallucinations take this feeling and amplify it.

☆ ☆ ☆

The term 'hypnopompic hallucination' was coined by Frederic W.H. Myers, a key member of the Society for Psychical Research. This organisation was founded in 1882 after discussions at a conference at the British National Association of

Spiritualists' headquarters in London. The mission of its members was to investigate aspects of the supernatural and psychic phenomena, with a view to gaining cohesive proof as to whether or not such things as telepathy, hauntings, and hypnotism really existed. Myers was a member of the founding committee of the Society, and produced a vast number of lectures, experiments and treatises until his death in 1901. Myers describes hypnopompic hallucinations in an essay published in 1892 in the *Proceedings of the Society for Psychical Research*, simply titled, 'The Subliminal Consciousness'. Much of the essay looks at pseudo-scientific phenomena such as telepathy and automatic writing. He hypothesises that 'the stream of consciousness in which we habitually live is not the only consciousness which exists in connection with our organism', and that our minds consist of layers of personality – some of which come to the surface during certain states of sleep or hypnosis.[5]

Further in the article, Myers turns his attention to the subliminal consciousness in dreams. He argues that the vivid and fantastical nature of dreams attests to his theory that there are deeper levels of consciousness with the power to create complex imitations of reality. The 'occasional prolongation of dream figures' into waking sight is proof of this – these hallucinations show that the brain can conjure images as intense and vivid as anything we might see in our waking lives. In naming this phenomenon, he tentatively suggests the term '*hypnopompic* illusions'. He relates the label directly to Alfred Maury's 1848 coinage of 'hypnagogic'; 'hypno' is the Greek for sleep, and where 'gogic' means to 'enter into', 'pompic' means to 'send away'. In other words, hypnopompic hallucinations are a phenomenon that occurs when our brain moves away from the state of sleep. I wonder how he would feel to know his term is still used today.

Despite framing the introduction to the term in a pseudo-scientific context, Myers accurately theorised the phenomenon as a projection of dream images onto waking sight. He continued to research hypnopompic hallucinations, bringing popularity to the term a decade later when he published his mammoth two-volume manuscript, *Human Personality and its Survival of Bodily Death*. Here, he notes that hallucinations are 'probably the highest point which man's visualising faculty ever reaches', and he even expresses a little jealousy towards those who experience this phenomenon, when he finds his own ability to visualise somewhat lacking.[6]

While there is certainly evidence to show that sleep-related hallucinations can be exacerbated by illness (I've had some truly spectacular nights when suffering from flu), they are not necessarily caused by any sort of morbid condition. In fact, Myers seems to want to celebrate hypnopompic hallucinations; they are a glimpse into how vivid the imagination can be. I can share Myers' fascination with this parasomnia, but I suspect he never threw his pillow across the room to shake off a phantom spider, or pulled a muscle in his arm while trying to fight off a shadowy figure. My imagination isn't always kind to me.

But hallucinations of this sort were described in medical essays and treatises long before Myers gave them a name. Despite not assigning them a specific term, French physician and psychiatrist Alexandre Brierre de Boismont illustrates them clearly in his 1853 text, *On Hallucinations: A History and Explanation, or, Apparitions, Visions, Dreams, Ecstasy, Magnetism and Somnambulism* (translated by Robert T. Hulme in 1859).

'The illusions of sleep,' he writes, 'may, like the hallucinations, continue at the moment of waking up, and even during the state of complete wakefulness, and may give rise to extravagant, criminal, and dangerous acts. Soon, however, the images of the night are diminished in intensity and disappear, and the person is amongst the first to be astonished at the language he has held, although he declares that at the time his sensations seemed to him to be perfectly natural.'[7] These strange acts, he notes, often occur in people who are otherwise in good mental health. He includes a particularly interesting case:

A young lady saw the wall open, and from the aperture there emerged a death's head, which placed itself upon a skeleton, and at the same time advanced towards her. Satisfied that this apparition was an illusion, she would reason with herself and endeavour to allay her fears: the matter terminated by her waking up.

This sounds very much like a hypnopompic hallucination, especially in the threatening way in which the skeleton approached her. I'm intrigued by the way that this woman had somehow learned to rationalise her sleep hallucinations; perhaps they happened so often that she could no longer be fooled into fearing what she saw. I can understand how she might have done it, since there are times when I doubt the reality of what I'm seeing. Largely, though, my hypnopompic hallucinations trigger my survival instincts. My brain becomes a primal mess of alarm bells, and I don't have the time or the mental capacity to calm down and explain the vision away. I know that this has happened to me before, but the sensation of being fully awake and rational only

makes the experience more terrifying to me. If I'm able to rationalise and tell myself that what I'm seeing isn't real, then why the
hell is it still here? I would love to able to talk to the woman of
Brierre de Boismont's anecdote, and find out how she faced a
vision of death itself and still managed to keep her cool. But anyway, it's comforting to know that she managed to do it. Maybe
I'll be able to dismiss my hallucinations just as easily, too.

Even earlier, in 1813, a Scottish physician named John
Ferriar published *An Essay Towards a Theory of Apparitions.*
Seeking to shed light on 'spectral delusions', Ferriar offers some
explanations of hallucinations.[8] He writes:

> When the brain is partially irritated, the patient fancies
> that he sees spiders crawling over his bed-cloths, or per-
> son; or beholds them covering the roof and walls of his
> room. If the disease increases, he imagines that persons
> who are dead, or absent, flit round his bed; that animals
> croud into his apartment, and that all these apparitions
> speak to him. These impressions take place, even while
> he is convinced of their fallacy. All this occurs some-
> times, without any degree of delirium.

Spiders, it seems, are a common shape for hypnopompic hallucinations to take form. I wish it could be something nice like
a puppy or a flower, but I suppose they don't really lend themselves to the imagery of night-time anxieties. In a way, I find it
quite heartening to read that I'm experiencing the same thing
as Ferriar's patients, two hundred years later. By a 'partially irri-
tated' brain, Ferriar is referring not to insanity but to anxiety,
fear, depression or a temporary illness that may include a fever.

But, as we saw in Flavie Waters' research, what later psychologists and neurologists demonstrate is that hypnopompic hallucinations often occur in mentally healthy people.

Interestingly, Ferriar uses his theories of hallucinations to try to explain away the belief in ghosts. He says that by 'accurately' examining such stories of horror and the supernatural, the 'appearance of a ghost would be regarded in its true light, as a symptom of bodily distemper, and of little more consequence than the head-ach and shivering attending a common catarrh.' Furthermore, he suggests that a person already prone to nighttime hallucinations can be adversely affected by a change of place. In other words, a night spent in a new bed could conjure up a hypnopompic hallucination of a phantom.

☆　☆　☆

An unfamiliar bed can sometimes encourage phantoms to appear. I remember staying over at a friend's house when I was a teenager. She lived in a very rural area, in a house on a narrow lane without any kind of street lighting. It was an old, quirky house with a peculiar layout of surprise staircases and hallways, and when we went to sleep the room was far darker than I normally experienced. I woke up in the middle of the night – my eyes just about able to pick out the shapes in her bedroom – and saw the silhouette of a person standing very still in the corner. I stared at the shape for a few moments, then shrugged and went back to sleep.

This was shortly after I met Meredith. I had already started to hallucinate spiders, which is perhaps why I didn't assume that this thing in my friend's house was something supernatural. But say I had never experienced hypnopompic hallucinations before, or only small things very rarely, and the first time I saw the image of a person was when I was staying in an old hotel. In that circumstance, I might wonder if I had actually seen a ghost.

Ghost stories take on a different meaning if you read them with sleep disorders and hallucinations in mind. Frequently, such stories occur at night and in the bedroom. Think of Ebenezer Scrooge in Charles Dickens' *A Christmas Carol*, visited by ghosts as he passes a fitful sleep on Christmas Eve. Ghost stories – particularly Victorian ones – favour the bedchamber. It was not simply a place of sleep, but also a place of sickness (often endured under a cocktail of strong medicines) and even death. On a thematic level, the veil between life and death was thin in the bedroom. Perhaps hypnopompic hallucinations, in this case, created a kind of vicious cycle. Stories about ghostly bedroom encounters might have fuelled night-time anxieties, and the dread of seeing a ghost might have provoked hallucinations of people.

An example of a possible hypnopompic hallucination being reported as a ghost can be found in novelist Catherine Crowe's 1848 non-fiction text, *The Night Side of Nature, or, Ghosts and Ghost Seers*. Crowe describes a spooky encounter experienced by fellow author Elizabeth Eastlake. While in St Petersburg, Russia, Eastlake spent the night in the house of a friend. 'No one who knows her,' writes Crowe, 'can suspect her of seeing spectral illusions, or being incapable of distinguishing her own condition when she saw anything whatever.'[9] Nevertheless, a spectral illusion is exactly what she saw that night.

She was woken up by a woman in Russian dress, who very gently and pleasantly – but without using words – urged her to get out of bed. Eastlake checked the time on her pocket-watch, and saw with confusion that it was only four o'clock in the morning. She showed the time to the woman, and then went back to sleep.

When, a few hours later, Eastlake got out of bed and went for breakfast, she asked her friend about the woman who'd been a little too eager to wake her up. Of course, the friend replied that there was no other woman in the house and dismissed her story as a dream. Eastlake, however, remained adamant that what she had seen was unquestionably real. 'The thing has ever remained utterly inexplicable,' says Crowe, and leaves the matter there.

Did Eastlake see a ghost, or was it a hypnopompic hallucination? Most of the time, my visions are terrifying, but not always. Sometimes they fascinate me, or I simply ignore them and roll over in bed. Eastlake didn't hear the woman come in, and only woke up when she was standing at her bedside. Although Eastlake perceived herself as awake, it sounds as though she had some confusion or delusion regarding the time. The fact that, despite being woken up by a strange woman at a strange hour, Eastlake was able to slip back into sleep suggests that she was in the half-awake state so favourable to hypnopompic hallucinations.

But hypnopompic hallucinations aren't purely image-based. Sometimes they occur as sounds. In 1705, an English physician and geologist named John Beaumont published *An Historical, Physiological and Theological Treatise of Spirits, Apparitions, Witchcrafts, and Other Magical Practices*. It contains hundreds of anecdotes collected from antiquity and from Beaumont's acquaintances and personal experiences. Beaumont relates his own stories with the certainty that they are otherworldly in source. He calls them his 'Spiritual Visitations', and writes about them with more pride than fear. Nevertheless, the stories sound remarkably like frequent experiences of hypnopompic hallucinations.

'For some Weeks together,' Beaumont writes, 'every Night, as soon as I was in Bed, a Spirit came with a little Bell Ringing in my Ear, and a Voice always Talking to me ...'[10]

Experiencing hypnopompic hallucinations as sounds is quite common. It happens to me often enough that I don't take notice of them in the same way I do their visual form. I will hear my Dad rattling the cat's metal dish, even though I'm a hundred miles away in Aberystwyth. I might catch the final trill of a landline phone I don't own, or I'll hear the beeping scanner of the postwoman about to deliver a phantom parcel at three in the morning. It's always domestic or everyday noises, quite boring and forgettable in comparison to the other things that happen to me at night. But they can sound incredibly vivid, and it's the way in which they seem to be external – something *heard*, not thought or imagined – that can disorient and confuse a sleeper.

Auditory sleep hallucinations were the subject of a study in 2011, conducted by Lourence L. Lewis-Hanna and his team at the University of Sheffield.[11] Again, similarities were drawn between hypnopompic hallucinations and schizophrenia – both share some characteristics of experiencing vivid sensory phenomena. But as Lewis-Hanna illustrates, sleep-related aural hallucinations produce only simple sounds such as a name or a ringing doorbell, whereas schizophrenia involves much more complex sentences. Lewis-Hanna's team focused solely on the former. They conducted a study of 100 participants, split into two groups depending on whether they experienced auditory sleep hallucinations or not. The focus was to gauge if auditory sensitivity affected participants' propensity for hearing imaginary sounds in their sleep. The data suggests that this is indeed the case; brain scans of the 'hallucinator group' showed enhanced stimulation in the brain in response to external sounds. In other words, they found that this form of hallucination doesn't necessarily have a pathological cause – it can simply be a matter of your sensitivity to noises.

☆ ☆ ☆

Towards the end of the nineteenth century, interest in hallucinations was becoming increasingly strong. This was, in part, due to the work of the Society for Psychical Research, and especially the research of F.W.H. Myers. The Society looked at hallucinations from two very different perspectives. On one hand, they were at the forefront of research into the physiological causes and conditions of hallucinations. On the other, they vigorously pursued the idea that hallucinations were a product of supernatural forces such as telepathy or visitations from spirits. Nevertheless, they consistently held discussions in their meetings and publications as to the true nature of hallucinations.

In 1886, Myers, together with fellow Society members Edmund Gurney and Frank Podmore, published an extensive study of hallucinations, spectres, and unexplained things seen by the human eye. It was called *Phantasms of the Living*, and it laid the foundations for some of their subsequent investigations. What they wanted to do in this book was to provide case studies and examine them in a rational, scientific manner in order to find the anecdotes that might truly have some sort of psychic or supernatural origin. They were particularly interested in 'thought-transference' – a psychic occurrence in which two living people send a message or vision to each other through the power of their mind. The most frequent 'cases' of this involved one person seeing another when the other was in grave danger or at death's door.

Later in the book, the men turn their attention to the hallucinations of sleep. They make it clear that many things seen when falling asleep or waking up are perfectly natural, despite how it feels at the time. However, there are a few anecdotes presented to them that they aren't so sure about, and they wonder if these might belong to their folder of evidence for 'thought-transference'. Here's an example from Mrs L.H. Saunders:

> Towards morning of the 10th January, 1885, I was conscious of a young woman standing by my bedside clad in a grey dressing gown, holding in her arms, towards me, a child. The woman was weeping bitterly, and said, 'Oh! Mrs Saunders, I am in such trouble.' I instantly recognised her as Mrs C.R. Seymour, and was about to interrogate her as to her trouble, when I was awakened by my husband asking me what was the matter, as I seemed so distressed.[12]

Mrs Saunders was so upset by this dream that she decided to write to Mrs Seymour's mother. She made the rather odd decision to tell the mother of her vision, and since Mrs Seymour lived far away in New Zealand, it had the effect of spreading panic through the family. A few months later, Mrs Saunders asked the mother if she had had any news. The mother said yes, but the news wasn't good. Mrs Seymour's daughter, Dottie, had recently died. It's a tragic story in any case, but what follows is a strange collection of corroborating statements, letters and dates providing 'complete confirmation' that what Mrs Saunders saw was a psychic vision from Mrs Seymour herself.

The men's interest in hallucinations reached a peak in the final decade of the nineteenth century, when they decided to take their discussions out into the public. Three years after the publication of *Phantasms of the Living*, in 1889, the Society for Psychical Research began a five-year study, called the Census of Hallucinations, in order to discover the frequency and nature of hallucinations in a large number of people. Their objective in the study was to 'ascertain what percentage of persons have had sensory hallucinations while awake, and not suffering from delirium or insanity', and to record a full description of the participants' experience.[13] In 1894, the Society published its report, which contains pages and pages of data and transcribed anecdotes collected over the course of the survey.

The Census was built around one main inquiry: 'Have you ever, when believing yourself to be completely awake, had a vivid impression of seeing or being touched by a living being or inanimate object, or of hearing a voice; which impression, so far as you could discover, was not due to any physical cause?'

Out of 17,000 respondents, the Society received 2,272 affirmative answers. When probing further into these respondents' experiences, they offered criteria such as 'Immediately after waking' – the very condition in which hypnopompic hallucinations occur. The Society was often torn between scientific inquiry and supernatural investigation. In the case of the Census, the Society was more interested in the hallucinations that could be interpreted as having paranormal causes, rather than those with more obvious neurological roots. Throughout the report, the writers mention their disregard of any anecdotes of hallucinations caused by sleep because they are too easily explained. Nevertheless, they still include the data and the transcripts of participants' experiences.

The report is engrossing to read, particularly the anecdotes. There are several that seem to be obvious hypnopompic hallucinations. For example, the report includes the response of Miss M.H.M., given in February 1890:

About fifteen years ago, I had gone to sleep without knowing it, a fire burning opposite the foot of my bed. Thinking I was awake, I thought I saw standing before my fire, at the right hand side, looking into it, with her back turned to me, so that I could not see her face, an elderly woman, rather stout, and dressed like an old-fashioned nurse or housekeeper, in a black cap tied close round the ears, and a large-checked shawl. The check was about four inches square, and black, pink, white and grey, the pink squares being specially distinct. Wondering what she was doing there, I sat up in bed to look at her, and the action of doing so woke me. I was fully conscious of suddenly waking, fully conscious that I had been asleep, and had awoken with a shock, yet I still saw the woman distinctly, with my eyes open and wide awake. She faded gradually. My heart beat for a moment; but I thought it was only the impression of a dream still remaining in my brain that appeared to be seen with my eyes. So I lay down and went to sleep again, and saw no more.

Motifs of death, decay, and Gothic imagery occur again and again throughout the Census responses. Not only was life expectancy much shorter and infant mortality much higher in Victorian Britain than it is today (Victorian novelists teach us that having the window open a bit too long means certain expiration), but popular culture was rife with images of skeletons, rotting corpses, and tombstones. The 'memento mori' (Latin for 'remember you are mortal' – cheery) was an object or token, ranging from a crudely carved coffin to elaborate dioramas and clocks depicting anything from an anatomy lesson to some sort of skeleton disco. These could be carried around with people as an everyday item – cufflinks, a pocket-watch – or proudly displayed on mantelpieces and in living rooms. The wonderful Wellcome Collection in London has a vast display of memento mori, and their collection is so large that some of it is also displayed in the Science Museum's Medicine Gallery, including Charles Darwin's whalebone walking stick topped with a skeletal head, eyes glowing with green glass. In the present day, these icons only emerge at Halloween, but in the nineteenth century they were ubiquitous.

It's no wonder, then, that visions of death and decay appear so often in the Census anecdotes. Perhaps this is part of what the nineteenth-century art critic John Ruskin meant when he talked about the 'evil eye'. To be evil-eyed, Ruskin says, is to 'have darkness in *us*, portable, perfect, and eternal.'[14] I like this idea, that my hallucinations draw from some kind of dark well inside me made up of bad experiences, worries, and the scary iconography and fiction I've encountered throughout my life. Do they go back into that well once I see them, or, to extend the metaphor even further, are they then 'exorcised'? Will there come a point where I stop hallucinating, because there's nothing left to scare me? It won't be for a while, anyway – the anecdotes in the Census have certainly given me fodder for future spooks. Miss E.A., for example, decided to grace the Society with this utterly horrifying story:

> I saw a figure standing by my bed. I had been awake some time. It was a summer morning, about 5 o'clock, and I saw the figure quite distinctly. It was tall and dressed in something grey, falling in long folds. The face was kind and I was not frightened at first, but it suddenly changed and the whole figure and face, as it were, fell to pieces in the most ghostly manner and vanished. I was about 22. It must be nine years since it [happened].

But what's especially interesting, and perhaps quite sad, too, is that a lot of the anecdotes with a supernatural or ghostly element feature family members. Mrs L.H.'s anecdote immediately follows that of Miss E.A., but presents a very different sort of morbid vision:

> I think the vision that I am about to describe occurred in March, 1891. I was asleep, when I woke with a start, it then being early morning. On looking round the room, I distinctly saw the head of a skeleton floating in the air, about a foot from the ceiling. I gazed at it intently (being now quite awake), when I saw it gradually change to my mother's head and face and float away, seemingly through the ceiling. My age [was] 35.

Sometimes the Census anecdotes involving departed loved ones are rather mild – the sleeper just sees them as they were in life. At other times, the hallucinated person is someone still alive, and when something grave *does* coincidentally happen to them, the hallucination is taken to be a premonition. In one sombre case, a man is keeping vigil through the night next to his young son who has just passed away – he sees a blue flame hovering over his son's body as though his soul had emerged out of him. Hallucinations can be frightening, but they can also provide comfort, too.

The Census demonstrated to the public the commonality of hallucinations. In amassing anecdotes from participants, it showed that people of all ages and backgrounds – and people without an underlying mental health problem – can experience illusory phenomena. It certainly generated more conversations about hallucinations, and helped to lift some of the stigma that associated hallucinations with insanity. The Society for Psychical Research is still going strong; perhaps one day they'll do a repeat of the Census. It would certainly be interesting to see how the content of our hallucinations has changed.

Over a hundred years after the Society's Census, a 2000 study by Maurice M. Ohayon showed that out of 13,057 participants of a hallucination survey, 38.7% had experienced some sort of hallucinatory episode. Of this percentage, 24.8% were thought to be hypnagogic hallucinations, and 6.6% had experienced a hypnopompic hallucination.[15] The 1894 report suggests that 2.5% of participants had experienced a hallucination either immediately upon waking or with the participant in bed – both of which are likely to lead to a hypnopompic hallucination – so it's interesting to see that there is some synchronicity between the studies, and that we may even be hallucinating a little more often (or that we're more willing to admit to it) in recent times.

☆ ☆ ☆

After I moved flats in July 2018, I thought I would be 'safe' from the woman I kept seeing in Aberystwyth. I'd never felt like that before – my hypnopompic hallucinations had never been consistent or bad enough for me to feel like another bed would be safer.

The hallucinations continued regardless. Back at my parents' house for the summer, in my bedroom, I woke up to a woman's disembodied head slowly turning into a teal-coloured tree trunk on the pillow next to me. Her face became long and cracked, and her mouth opened in a hollow and silent scream. For a few seconds, I knew it was my fault. I was thrown from abject horror to a sense of crushing guilt that I was responsible for what was happening to this woman's face.

The next night, I saw a man, or what was more like the shadow of a man, peering down at me. I couldn't see more of him than a silhouette, except for his eyes. His eyes were large and shining brighter than the moon outside. His head was misshapen; his cheeks were angular and asymmetrical, and his forehead bloomed outwards like a mushroom. I looked into his white eyes. His hands came up over me. The fear I felt then was like a thousand snakes writhing in my arms and legs. I swung my fists, I clawed at him, I kicked until the bed rocked. I was completely blind to all reason, and any part of me that knew the man wasn't real was drowned out by the impulse to fight. In fact, I was still fighting for a few moments after the figure had disappeared. It took a long time for me to calm down again. My hands trembled so badly that I couldn't unscrew the cap from the water bottle by my bed.

I don't recognise myself in my wild attempt to fight off whatever it is I can see. I'm quite a timid person; I wince if someone does a loud sneeze near me. When I was an undergraduate, one of my friendship group's favourite late-night conversations was our strategy for a zombie apocalypse. I couldn't picture myself doing anything my friends were suggesting – gather weapons, build a fortress in a warehouse, walk around with a flamethrower – so I decided my strategy would just be to lie down in the road and accept my fate. But my sleep has taught me that I'm not quite as cowardly as I think. If I was, then surely my reaction to these threatening hallucinations would be to scream for help or launch myself out of bed and try to get to the door. But I don't. I throw punches like a pint-sized Rocky Balboa, using strength and speed that I didn't think I had. And this, on top of my sleep-walking, is why I can't fall asleep if I'm not in a bed by myself.

Because I've been talking about my research and experiences quite openly for a few years, people sometimes tell me about their own hypnopompic hallucinations. Now that they know their experiences have a clinical name and aren't necessarily a sign of madness, they candidly tell me about what they've seen in the middle of the night. Hypnopompic hallucinations are still relatively unexplored; they either exist harmlessly on their own or are a small symptom of a much larger neurological disorder. There is no particular treatment for them. Earlier, I mentioned the work of Felicity Waite and the sleep disorders of her schizo-phrenia patients. Her team are developing methods of cognitive therapy to soothe nightmares and hypnopompic hallucinations.

For example, one technique uses a set of cue cards on the bedside table; when a patient wakes up to a hallucination, they can grab the cards and read through reassuring messages that attempt to explain and rationalise their experience. The main form of Waite's CBT is education: by telling patients about REM sleep and the induction of hypnopompic hallucinations, it will normalise and therefore lessen the effect of the phenomenon.

I hope that Waite's work will be used outside of the psychiatric hospital, too. From the conversations I have, the simple act of learning about hypnopompic hallucinations makes people less afraid and less secretive about their experiences. I suspect that if we had more discussions about these types of sleep disorders and how they can affect the general public, successful methods of support and education could be developed.

☆ ☆ ☆

Hypnopompic hallucinations can appear on their own, or as part of a much worse parasomnia: sleep paralysis. The demon squatting on the sleeper's chest has proliferated in fiction and culture for centuries, and continues to affect our sleep in the modern guise of alien abductions. In the next chapter, we will delve deeper into the night to encounter this deeply terrifying parasomnia.

Chapter 4

Hag-ridden

When I wake up in the middle of the night, I don't just see things that aren't real. Sometimes, it's a more complex delusion that involves more of my senses. In other words, I *feel* hallucinations, too.

A few years ago, I was having a distressing dream. I was standing outside, giving a talk to a boisterous crowd. Dozens of people were pressing too close to me, and I was struggling to raise my voice above the noise they were making. Scanning the faces, my attention suddenly snagged on one person in particular.

Where the rest of the crowd were animated and moving, one woman was standing absolutely still. I met her gaze, and the sight of her eyes chilled me – even remembering it now sets me on edge. Her eyes were uncannily large and bright white, almost glowing. The more she stared at me, the more terrified I became. All the while, the crowd was pushing against me, roaring in my ears. The anxiety dream became a full-blown nightmare, reaching a crescendo of noise while the woman continued to stare in threatening silence.

I woke up. I had rolled onto my front in my sleep, and the first thing I wanted to do was shift to my usual position on my right side. But I couldn't. I couldn't move. The lingering fear from my dream now erupted into panic. I was completely paralysed; I couldn't control even the tip of my finger.

And then, slowly, like melting ice, I realised that I wasn't simply paralysed: something was pinning me down.

A weight shifted on my back. Someone was on top of me. The woman from the dream. She was real, and she was here. I thought I had escaped her when I woke up but somehow she was here, with me, crushing me into my mattress.

I tried to scream, but my mouth wouldn't work. I tried to push her off, but she stayed put. Her weight was solid; I could feel her knees digging into the small of my back.

She shifted again, this time rolling off onto the mattress beside me. My head was turned to the right, and she had moved away to my left. I felt the mattress bend under her, and I knew if I looked over my shoulder, she would be there.

Seconds passed. Nothing happened, but I was still aware of her presence next to me. But I found I could twitch my fingers, then move my hands, and eventually I risked a quick peek at the other side of my bed.

There was nothing.

Of course there was nothing. I switched on the light, and patted down the crinkled sheet where I had convinced myself the woman was lying. It was cold. Then I swore at myself for even checking, for allowing myself yet again to be convinced of intruders in my bedroom. But I had *felt* her knees in my back, as sure as I could now feel my hands angrily rubbing my face. Not only that, but the mattress moved under her weight – how had I hallucinated that?

This is the phenomenon known as sleep paralysis. I started experiencing this only a few years ago, but it now happens to me several times a month. According to Shelley Adler, in their 2011 book *Sleep Paralysis: Night-Mares, Nocebos and the Mind-Body Connection*, around 25–30% of people experience sleep paralysis at least once in their lifetime.[1]

Nothing else I go through at night baffles or scares me quite as much as this; it's the way I often feel, very vividly, hands around my wrists, ankles and neck. The sensation of a stranger's skin against mine, just for a few moments, is so unmistakably real that I can often still feel it for the rest of the day. Usually, what happens to me at night doesn't affect me during the day. With sleep paralysis, however, I find I'm tense for a long time afterwards. I'll feel queasy and my skin will prickle; if a particular part of me was 'touched', usually my neck, an uncomfortable pressure will linger like a ghost.

☆　☆　☆

When we dream, during our REM phase of sleep, our brain does in fact send directions to the muscles based on what we see ourselves doing. If we are dreaming about playing tennis, messages will be sent to the arm as though we're swinging our racquet to meet the ball. Obviously, there are many reasons why this could cause a problem. In order to negate this potential chaos, the brain *also* paralyses the body. It can then send all the signals it likes to our muscles based on what we're dreaming about, but the muscles won't move. REM disorder is when this paralysis doesn't work, and it can lead to awful consequences. Sleep paralysis, on the other hand, is when you partly wake up before the paralysis has naturally worn off. But because you're still in a dreamlike state, your brain conjures up something to explain the sensation of pressure on your chest and limbs. You see monsters, and you are at their mercy.

The way this type of hallucination involves *all* the senses, and tricks them so well, is enough to convince anyone that what they're experiencing is real. It's no surprise, then, that historical representations of this parasomnia are riddled with demons and dark magic. While it is much better understood now, it used to be closely aligned with witchcraft in particular.

☆ ☆ ☆

Various names have been given to sleep paralysis in the past, and most of them are aligned with supernatural forces. The old name for sleep paralysis was 'nightmare' – a word that has now come to mean a bad dream or a generally troubled sleep. The word 'mare' comes from *mara*, an Old Norse word for a witch who would lie on people's chests and try to suffocate them.[2] It was also associated with a horse, possessed by witchcraft, that would come and trample the sleeper. When the episode had a sexual aspect to it, it was sometimes described as a demonic 'incubus' when taking a male form, or 'succubus' when female. Other names included being 'hag-ridden' or suffering from 'wizard-pressing' (my personal favourite – I think we need to bring this term back). These names encouraged supernatural interpretation, and further heightened the fear of witchcraft and the devil that was prevalent around Europe up to the seventeenth century.

But as Europeans colonised other parts of the world, they brought their superstitions with them. Particularly in America, the English Puritans who settled there created an environment of religious anxiety over who would be saved by God, and who would be eternally damned. Some of the most infamous cases of widespread terror of witchcraft in America are the Salem Witch Trials. These deadly court cases began in 1692 in the small, devoutly Puritan village of Salem, Massachusetts. Here, fear of constant temptation and corruption by the devil pervaded the imagination, and women were seen as particularly liable to fall from God's grace. In February 1692, two young girls, Betty Parris and Abigail Williams, began to behave erratically. They said they were being pricked by needles, though no physical injuries could be seen, and started to have 'fits' of screaming, violence, and convulsions. Other girls in the village – Ann Putnam and Elizabeth Hubbard – followed with similar symptoms, and the situation in Salem soon snowballed into a fatal occurrence of mass hysteria.

In an attempt to get to the bottom of the girls' ailments, older women in the village were accused of bewitching and cursing the children. It seems strange that the accusations would be taken seriously, but as Marian L. Starkey explains, religious belief surrounding the trials accepted that the devil didn't necessarily leave physical evidence behind him, and as such, 'hallucinations, dreams, and mere fancies' could be used as proof in court.[3] The trials began in earnest, with the first including Sarah Good, Sarah Osborne, and a slave from South America known as Tituba. It seemed as though everyone was pointing a finger at someone else, accusing them of witchcraft and being in league with the devil, and the rumours and reports became ever more outlandish. In the end, over two hundred accusations had been made, and nineteen people were executed by hanging.

The trial archives are currently accessible online via the Virginia Library, and they're worth having a look at. There are maps, letters, court transcripts and images pertaining to the trials and the community. What strikes me is just how frequently sleep paralysis is described in the accusations.

A particularly interesting document is that of the court case between Richard Coman and Bridget Bishop on 2 June 1692. Bishop was the first to be killed in the trials, and much of the testimony against her features descriptions remarkably similar to the experience of sleep paralysis. This case is one such example.

Coman says that Bishop and two other women appeared in his bedroom one night and 'lay upon [his] Breast ... and soe oppressed him that he could not speake nor stur noe not so much as to awake his wife althow he Endeavered much soe to do itt.'[4] The paralysis occurred again the following Saturday night, in which Coman felt himself grabbed by the throat and lifted out of bed. He told his wife, who advised him to sleep with his sword by him. Sure enough, he saw Bridget and the women again. This time, he tried to call out to his wife but was 'Immediatly strook speechless & could not move hand or foote and Immediatly they gott hold of my sword & strived to take it from mee but I held soe fast as thay could not gett it away.'

Eight days following this testimony, Bridget Bishop was executed for witchcraft.

What's important, and quite frustrating, to realise is that 1692 is rather late in terms of witchcraft beliefs. Much of what had previously been understood as having supernatural causes, namely diseases and unexplained death, was already being described in much more realistic terms. Reginald Scot, a sixteenth-century English politician, wrote *The Discoverie of*

Witchcraft in 1584. Its title suggests that Scot stumbled in on a gathering of spellcasters, but its purpose is quite the opposite: throughout the text, Scot outlines the natural causes for many phenomena thought to be the result of witches. This isn't to say Scot didn't believe in *any* supernatural force; he was a Protestant, and despite his scepticism of witchcraft, he still fervently believed in God's power. Stories of witchcraft, though, were for Scot nothing more than a result of illness or disturbed perception. One of his topics in *The Discoverie of Witchcraft* is the superstition of the incubus. He describes the phenomenon as follows:

> But in truth, this Incubus is a bodilie disease (as hath been said) although it extend unto the trouble of the mind: which of some is called The mare, oppressing manie in their sleepe so sore, as they are not able to call for helpe, or stir themselves under the burthen of that heavie humor, which is ingendered of a thicke vapour proceeding from the cruditie and rawnesse in the stomach: which ascending up into the head oppresseth the brain, in so much as manie are much infeebled thereby, as being mightilie haunted therewith.[5]

Scot emphasises the bodily causes of sleep paralysis. While he wasn't correct in describing its origin as a digestive issue, he was certainly closer to the mark than thinking it was caused by witchcraft. This text was published over a hundred years before the Salem Witch Trials, demonstrating just how long it took for the suspicion of witchcraft to be overtaken by contemporary ideas of rationalism.

The cures for sleep paralysis mirrored the shift in belief from the supernatural to the scientific. Before the birth of rationalism, there was a definite sense of needing magic to fight magic. One of the most popular forms of protection against the *mara* were rocks and minerals thought to have been formed by supernatural means. 'Mare-stanes' were almost perfectly circular rocks with an eroded centre – a bit like a doughnut – formed in fast-flowing parts of rivers. An article in *The Journal of the Anthropological Institute of Great Britain and Ireland* describes three mare-stanes collected by Lord Ducie in 1887, and demonstrates the variety of local folklore regarding these objects. The first, chillingly, had human teeth fixed in the stone's holes. These could be hung up in stables, tied to a stable key or around a horse's neck to stop witches from riding off with them to stomp on sleeping victims' chests. How exactly this was supposed to work seems to have been lost to time; as noted in the discussion, 'But in what manner a stone with a hole in it sufficed to exclude witches, or how the nightmare was transferred to the human being, involved more difficult questions.'[6] A similar talisman was the 'thunder stone', a smooth, bullet-shaped rock that was believed to be thunder captured and solidified. These are actually belemnites, the fossilised tentacles of a prehistoric squid commonly found on beaches in the UK. I'm a big fan of all things dinosaur- and fossil-related, so I do in fact own a few belemnites. They definitely don't work for me.

But as the understanding of sleep paralysis moved towards a physical, rather than supernatural cause, it was thought that it could be prevented or cured by lifestyle changes and medicinal remedies. For a long time, really until we knew about REM and the stages of sleep, sleep paralysis was chalked up as a result of overindulgence in food. Heavy, rich, or bad food late in the evening was thought to lie on the stomach and produce the sensation of weight on the chest and any accompanying hallucinations. This is why, in Charles Dickens' *A Christmas Carol*, Ebenezer Scrooge's first thought when supernatural events begin to occur is that he shouldn't have eaten cheese before bed. When the ghost of Jacob Marley appears in Scrooge's bedroom, he seems a little disappointed that he isn't as spooky as expected. Scrooge explains that he doesn't believe Marley is real, that his senses are playing tricks on him:

> 'Why do you doubt your senses?'
> 'Because,' said Scrooge, 'a little thing affects them. A slight disorder of the stomach makes them cheats. You may be an undigested bit of beef, a blot of mustard, a crumb of cheese, a fragment of an underdone potato. There's more of gravy than of grave about you, whatever you are!'[7]

Ho-ho. I might have to try that line myself. But in all seriousness, food was considered to be the main cause of any kind of upset sleep. In my travels through old treatises, a rumour pops up on occasion: allegedly, the famous Gothic novelist Ann Radcliffe, who wrote some of the earliest novels of that movement, such as *The Mysteries of Udolpho* (1794), deliberately ate raw steak to make herself ill and provoke inspiration through wild dreams and hallucinations.

Ways to prevent and cure sleep paralysis as a bodily affliction included eating lighter meals or taking a purgative if a person felt that they had eaten too much. It wasn't believed to be purely the fault of bad food, however. William Hammond, MD, in his 1869 book, *Sleep and its Derangements*, says he has 'known it be caused by the collar of the night-gown being too tight, and by the pillow being under the head and not under the shoulders, thus putting the head at such an angle with the body as to constrict the blood-vessels of the neck, and by the head falling over the side of the bed.'[8] Hammond also recommends the 'uniformly successful' potassium bromide, with doses of between twenty and forty grains three times a day. Potassium bromide was a popular medicine in the nineteenth century, used mostly to treat epilepsy and as a sedative. It's now only used in veterinary medicine, and isn't approved for human consumption.

☆ ☆ ☆

Nothing reminds me of Meredith quite like sleep paralysis. Even though my encounters with her were never explicitly physical, there is something about the feeling of sleep paralysis – being under the control of a sinister figure looming over me, the sensation of being suffocated, of being pinned down – that makes my stomach squirm in exactly the same way it did when I was fifteen.

Not all of my sleep paralysis experiences involve Meredith, but I am certain I wouldn't have sleep paralysis at all if not for her. I seem to have two types: one is a heavy, demonic attack, the other is more subtle and 'handsy'. I'm not sure which one is worse.

I remember Meredith's hands quite distinctly. I think it's because I felt so awkward and uncomfortable that I fixated on them, rather than have to look at her looking at me. She had incredibly sharp, pointed nails and huge rings on almost every finger. She would pat me a lot, like I was a toddler or a small dog.

Little pats on the head or a hand on my shoulder or upper arm. She would also make fun of the way I pushed my glasses up my nose, mirroring me with her hand and chuckling every time I did it until I stopped wearing my glasses altogether. In another way, though, my own hands began to bother me. The stress of being with her erupted in some of the worst eczema I've ever experienced. Still mostly clueless as to why I felt so uncomfortable all that year, I chalked it up to my GCSEs. I developed a nervous habit of scratching my elbows, and by the time summer came I was in agony – my hands were both a saviour and my own worst enemy, and my elbows were ringed in fire and caked in cool, blessed E45 cream.

Once I had moved to a separate college, Meredith became a little bolder.

On one occasion when I was about eighteen, I was standing in front of her while we talked. As usual, she was in my personal space. Being older now, and not quite as naive, I had started my years-long battle to try to separate myself from her. I began to see a nasty side to her; she would always tell me how people 'betrayed' her, and that she 'would never recover' if I upset her too. She'd say over and over again that she was always there for me, but ignored me when I actually came to her for help. Sometimes, though, more at the beginning of it all before she knew me better, she was kind and encouraging and paid attention to me in the way all teenagers crave. I think I always wanted to find that part of her again, so whenever she wanted to meet, I went. I used to hate myself for this, but with a bit of distance I can understand why – after all, she actively wanted me to be in a position where I was excited to see her. At this point, while I still came running, it was like looking at the aftermath of a car crash – I didn't want to be there, I *knew* I shouldn't be there, but I couldn't stop myself.

It was with this torn feeling, of hoping for kindness but preparing to run, that I stood before her that evening. I can't remember what we were talking about, just the initial polite questions of a catch-up conversation, but she suddenly paused mid-sentence. She reached over and clamped her hands on my shoulders, pushing them down.

'You're too tense, Alice,' she said.

That moment, and the feeling of her fingers squeezing the bones of my shoulders, is often replayed as sleep paralysis. I wake up, not being able to move, and experiencing the sensation of fingers and hands all over me. Most of the time, the fingers focus on a few specific places: my ankles, my face, my hair, and around my neck. I don't see anything when this happens, but unless you've also experienced something similar it's hard to emphasise just how stomach-churning it feels. It isn't real, but it is to me. For that moment, her hands *are* there, pinching my stomach, pulling me down the mattress by my feet. There's a lot of personality and emotion in the way the fingers poke and press my skin. It's like being told something. Sometimes the hands are gentle and move slowly – a thumb grazing my cheek or smoothing down my wavy hair; on other nights, the hands want to hurt me. But regardless of what I feel the hands do, there's a sense of delight in my fear and paralysis. The hands are possessive. Even the softest brush of a hand on my face very clearly tells me that I am at the mercy of someone or something else.

The morning after, the hands seem to linger and I wear the experience like a heavy coat. I find myself brooding over what happened with Meredith, even if the sleep paralysis seemed far removed from those memories, and my heart beats quick and sharp like a startled lizard.

☆ ☆ ☆

Perhaps the most famous depiction of sleep paralysis is Henry Fuseli's 'The Nightmare', painted in 1781. In the painting, a woman is draped over a bed, her upper torso and head lolling over the side. There's no way to tell if she's asleep or dead. On her chest squats a little demon, face contorted in an ugly grimace. But he isn't looking at her, beautiful as she is; it's as though this is all in a night's work for the incubus, as though he's caused so many nightmares that the novelty has worn off. Behind the woman is a red curtain fading into the black of night. The curtain is parted, and through the gap pokes the head of a wild-eyed, demonic horse – the *mara*. This isn't the only Fuseli painting that deals with parasomnias, as we saw in Chapter 2, but it is his best-known.

The thing that draws me to this painting is the same thing that excites me about dream sequences in movies: it's all presented as real. The incubus and the horse are tangible, vivid objects in the painting. The woman's white gown and ghost-pale complexion arrests our attention, but then we take in the rest of the scene: the eye is drawn first to the demon on her chest, and then to the leering horse behind. Moreover, the woman isn't even looking at the monsters in her room; her eyes are shut. Instead, it is we ourselves, the spectators on the scene, who can see the demons of sleep. And perhaps more chillingly, the monsters are staring back. 'You're next,' the incubus seems to say. There's nothing hallucinatory about the picture. It's real.

There are a number of eighteenth- to twentieth-century medical treatises that focus on the incubus. What's interesting is that they are written by doctors and physicians who experience sleep paralysis themselves. A fascinating example is John Bond's *An Essay on the Incubus, Or Night-mare* (1753). Bond explains in the preface his mission for the book: he has suffered for many years with frequent episodes of sleep paralysis, but, as a physician, is disappointed by the lack of medical books and treatises on the subject. By exploring his own tortured nights with his medical eye, it seems as though he is trying to make himself less afraid.

Bond suggests that the incubus is experienced not from bad digestion, but from 'stagnation of the Blood'.[9] Throughout his treatise, Bond describes some rather extreme case studies that he has encountered during his career: a man who experienced sleep paralysis every night for two years until he died, a young woman who suffered the parasomnia in the form of a sexual assault and awoke to find blood gushing from her nose and mouth. He analyses these in the clipped tone of a Man of Science, offering criticism of their treatment and suggesting what would have been a better course of action. But he returns often to his own attacks of the incubus, his 'Monster of the night', and he fails to maintain the same tone of rationality that he held when discussing the anecdotes of others. At one point, he writes:

> I have been so much oppress'd by this enemy of rest, that I would have given ten thousand worlds like this for some Person that would either pinch, shake, or turn me off my Back; and I have been so much afraid of its intolerable insults, that I have slept in a chair all night,

rather than give it an opportunity of attacking me in an horizontal position.

Bond resorts to some rather extreme (read: don't try this at home) methods to cure himself of sleep paralysis. While he starts the treatise emphasising the relationship between blood and the incubus, he begins to follow some of the popular contemporary discourse regarding sleep paralysis and poor digestion. His treatment: drain yourself of all bodily fluids until you're a dry husk of a person, and then you'll have so many other health problems that sleep paralysis will be the least of your worries. He suggests bleeding by the technique of cupping – a method of cutting the skin, applying a glass bell jar over the wound, then drawing out the blood using a sickeningly large syringe. Bond describes how he experimented with this treatment. At first, he bled himself regularly. When he found that it had the opposite effect, that the incubus was 'aggravated rather than abated', he rather stubbornly decided to double-down on his method, drawing twenty ounces of blood instead of the usual eight or ten. But he then reduced this from every month to once a year, after which he declared himself cured. It feels like a somewhat unsatisfactory conclusion to Bond's otherwise gripping personal narrative; it's not clear exactly *how* his blood-letting practice stopped his encounters with the incubus, and Bond doesn't offer any further explanation.

☆　☆　☆

Sleep paralysis is a nightmare experienced through flesh. It feels so real that, while it's happening, no amount of rationalisation or research will convince you that it's all in your head. How *can* it be in your head, when you can feel every sharp bump of the demon's knees pressing into your stomach? Perhaps it's this ambiguity, of not being able to trust your senses and perceptions, that makes it difficult to talk about. Most of the stories we've encountered so far in this chapter frame sleep paralysis as something ghostly and supernatural. Even in medical treatises such as Bond's, there's an aspect of embellishment – as though, by leaning into the macabre imagery and wrapping the story in elements of the fantastic, it's easier to describe.

I used to pack up my sleep paralysis experiences into some dark recess of my brain, never to come out again. I suppose I felt like they might recur if I did talk about it – that I might coax it out of myself. Reading about other people's encounters with the *mara* makes me feel less isolated and strange. It's helpful to unpack these memories, to admit that they frightened us, and to drag these phantoms out into the light and see them for what they really are.

There's one particular episode of sleep paralysis that haunted me, and I never talked about it at the time. I now realise how much it would have helped to put it into words. It happened a couple of years ago; I had gone back to my parents' house for the Easter vacation. Often, the change in sleeping environment from my Aberystwyth flat to my childhood bedroom sparks a sudden flurry of strange nights. I think I sleep deeper when I'm back in my 'own' bed, at least for the first few days, and some of my most memorable (for better or worse) sleep phenomena have been during my visits home. On this occasion, my PhD was coming to an end, and I was just starting to think about the initial idea for this book. My sleep had been getting stranger recently, and I was being more reflective about it than usual.

I had been making some notes of what I felt and saw, writing down my dreams and any hallucinations. It was at this time when I discovered that keeping a dream diary seems to make my parasomnias worse. The dreams became more and more vivid the more I thought about them and turned them into a written narrative, and then I found I was having lucid dreams more often, and then hallucinating in the night. At first I thought it was great for generating material for the book, and I soldiered through the phantom spiders and Meredith dreams. But then this episode of sleep paralysis happened, and I abandoned my dream diary for a long time.

I dreamt I was looking at myself in my bedroom mirror. It was night, but the moon was bright and I could see the dim shape of myself. I moved my hand to my hair; my reflection moved its hand to its hair. I put my arm down again. There was a pause. My reflection put its arm down again, too.

I frowned. In the darkness, I saw a gleam in the mirror. My reflection was smiling.

My stomach lurched. Whatever I was looking at wasn't me. I was watching someone else move in my image. My reflection's smile grew and became a monstrous grimace, teeth flashing like knives in the moonlight. I felt my heart beat furiously in my chest, but I couldn't look away. I was fixed to the spot, and then I couldn't tell who was on the right side of the mirror. Was *I* the reflection, after all?

I woke up gasping for breath, staring up in horror at the ceiling.

A second later, I found that my body wouldn't move. I had, by then, experienced this situation a few times and I had foolishly got into a mindset that by doing enough reading, I'd be able to rationalise the demons away. I tried to calm myself down. I was only paralysed; nothing had happened yet, and that gave me a little breathing space to think about what I might experience and meet it head-on. *Next will come a hand on my ankle*, I thought, *and I won't be scared because I know it's not real.* If I could give the episode an air of predictability, then maybe it wouldn't happen at all.

But then I felt it: something *under* my skin. I had been waiting for the hands to seize me by the throat or the knobbly knees in my stomach, but I had not expected this. There was a demon attacking me from the *inside*. It felt thin, like razor-sharp ribbons sliding into incisions along my arms and legs, wrapping around my bones and weaving through my muscles, taking over. It didn't hurt, but it felt excruciating in a sick, violating way. It wasn't an assault, this time, but an intrusion. There was nothing I could do to fight back; I was becoming increasingly small inside my own body.

My shoulders began to twitch, but I was no longer able to control them. Whatever it was that was now coiled around my bones was moving for me. There was an overwhelming sense of weightlessness and I was forced upwards like a jack-in-the-box. And then I started to tip forwards. Just before I fell head-first to the floor, I felt the tight grip of the intruder dissolve. There was a rush like the wind in an Underground station, and I found myself staring at the ceiling again. I blinked a few times, and tentatively lifted my fingers one by one. I moved my ankles, drew my knees up. I was back in my own body.

After a few moments, I calmed down enough to know the experience for what it really was. But it left me deeply unsettled. It was unlike anything I had ever felt, sleep paralysis or otherwise. I had been so convinced that I was being possessed, that something was crawling underneath my skin and I was being swallowed up inside my skull. How the hell did my brain come up with something like that? How did it make the sensation feel so real?

☆ ☆ ☆

Sleep paralysis, when it occurs, takes mostly a demonic form. The strange sensation of being unable to move elicits fear in us, and that fear conjures up images of ghosts, skeletons, witches and monsters. Sometimes it can be an erotic or pleasant experience, too, though the imagination still likes to warp and twist it somehow. A chilling example of this is found in S.W. Langston Parker's *On the Effects of Certain Mental and Bodily States Upon the Imagination* (1876). It's one of those anecdotes that made me do a little internal scream when I first read it, so I thought it was very necessary to share.

> I remember the case of a gentleman who experienced an attack of nightmare soon after the death of his wife, produced by supping at a late hour of some unwholesome food. She died soon after their marriage, the attachment preceding which had been long and ardent. He imagined that she was restored to him from the dead, and, like the Eurydice of Orpheus, was not tainted by the damps or dishonours of the grave – the demon of Corruption had not dared to lay a finger upon her sainted form, but she was, to his imagination, gay and blooming as she first appeared to him, a fair-haired girl, sporting

among the flowers her hand had planted, whose beauty was immeasurably inferior to her own: he clasped the delightful vision to his bosom, and once more dwelt in an Elysium of earthly happiness which, alas! was soon to be shadowed by the phantoms of icy despair. Suddenly, by one of those strange changes which are peculiar to the phenomena of our dreams, he was stretched upon the bed, and the phantom of his deceased wife seated upon his breast: her beauty began to fade, the skin to peel, and turn blue, the lip lost its vermilion and the eye its lustre, and he laboured in an agony of terror to throw off from his body the lifeless corpse, which, with a weight like that of Ossa and Pelion, appeared to be pressing him through the earth to her own clay tenement.[10]

The worst part of this anecdote is that, because of sleep paralysis, the man was afraid of his wife. Or at least, the image of his wife. Did this night tarnish the memory of her, I wonder? It makes me think of my own experiences, and how sleep paralysis can take an unpleasant but faded memory, or a person who wronged us a long time ago, and make it monstrous and fresh. With this anecdote in particular, it's also worth noting that Victorian culture delighted in all things morbid and horrible.

Funerals, post-mortem photography, mourning rituals and general reminders of mortality were incredibly prevalent in nineteenth-century society. The imagery of death and decay was everywhere, including the mantelpieces of a perfectly healthy family. As we've previously seen, a popular form of visualising death and mortality was through owning memento mori – small objects and ornaments featuring coffins or skeletons. A common type of memento mori is a half-and-half model of a human figure or head – one side is beautiful, with healthy, flushed cheeks and perfect hair, the other side is in a late stage of decay, a desiccated skeleton with bugs crawling over it. With images like these pervading the public imagination, it's no wonder that Langston Parker's man saw his wife change from angelic beauty to demonic corpse.

Ten years later, in 1886, members of the Society for Psychical Research published the influential book we encountered in the previous chapter, *Phantasms of the Living*. This multi-volume epic sought to investigate a number of strange and hallucinatory states, mostly with the idea of disproving (or finding concrete and irrefutable evidence for) notions of telepathy. Written by Edmund Gurney, F.W.H. Myers and Frank Podmore, *Phantasms of the Living* is not simply an interrogation of supposedly super-natural experiences, it's also a fantastic compilation of anecdotes pertaining to sleep-related phenomena.

Possibly my favourite anecdote in *Phantasms of the Living* is one of sleep paralysis. It was written in 1884 by Mrs Frances Lightfoot, who was, as the Society hilariously notes, 'none the worse witness because she takes not the slightest interest in our work.' It's fortunate that they thought so, because it's a skin-crawling read. This is Mrs Lightfoot's story:

> I had put aside my book, lowered the gas, and at a little after midnight I was sound asleep. As I knew afterwards, I must have slept about 3 hours, when I was suddenly aroused (and was, so far as I know, *perfectly wide awake*) by a violent noise at my door, which was locked. I have some recollection of feeling astonished (of fear I had

none) at seeing rather than hearing within the instant my door thrown violently open, as though by someone in great anger, and I was instantly conscious that someone, something – what shall I call *it*? – was in the room. For the hundredth part of a second it seemed to pause just within the room, and then by a movement, which it is impossible for me to describe – but it seemed to move with a rapid push – *it* was at the foot of my bed. Again a pause; for again the hundredth part of a second, and the figure-shape rose. I *heard* it, but as it got higher its movements quieted, and presently *it* was above my bed, lying horizontally, its face downwards, parallel with my face, its feet to my feet, but with a distance of some 3 or 4 feet between us. This for a moment, whilst I waited simply in astonishment and curiosity (for I had not the faintest idea of either who or what it was), but no fear, and then it spoke. In an instant I recognised the voice, the old familiar imperious way of speaking, as my Christian name sounded clear and full through the room. 'Frances,' it repeated, 'I want you; come with me. Come at once.' *My* voice responded as instantaneously, 'Yes, I'll come. What need for such a hurry?' and then came a quick imperative reply, 'But you must come *at once*; come instantly, without a moment's pause or hesitation.' I seemed to be drawn upwards by some extraordinary magnetic influence, and then just as suddenly and violently thrown down again.[11]

When the episode was over, Mrs Lightfoot described herself as having one thought 'simply burnt' into her mind: 'She is dead.'

The following day, while in conversation, the subject was brought to some mutual friends. When asked if Mrs Lightfoot had heard any news of a lady named Mrs Reed, Frances rather bluntly exclaimed that she was dead. It was Mrs Reed whom Frances believed had visited her in the night. However, no one had heard about this tragedy; in fact, when they did hear from the Reeds shortly afterwards, it was to report that Mrs Reed was much improved in her health. But, as Mrs Lightfoot so dramatically ends her tale, a month after her experience came news of the death of Mrs Reed.

Mrs Lightfoot seems to hide her superstition behind a staunch scepticism. She persists that she doesn't believe in such things as telepathy, yet there is clearly a part of her that wonders if Mrs Reed had actually sent her a message. On the other hand, she does refer to this experience as a 'dream', and Gurney, Myers and Podmore similarly describe it as a 'sensory hallucination'. It is, though, unmistakably sleep paralysis. The involvement of multiple senses, the sense of something approaching and looming over the sleeper, and, more importantly, that 'magnetic influence' – the sudden feeling of weightlessness before crashing back down – is a tell-tale feature of this parasomnia.

The death of Mrs Reed must be coincidental; her health was clearly in question. Frances frames the anecdote by saying that she often wrote to Mrs Reed, but that Mrs Reed's letters had dwindled recently. She was clearly worried about her friend, and this worry manifested itself in a complex episode of sleep paralysis.

What I like most about Mrs Lightfoot's story is its rich description and compelling narrative. It is written like a stereotypical ghost story, complete with its macabre revelation at the

end. This is what particularly fascinates me about the anecdotes of the Victorian era; there is something creative about
them. They are works of literature, so closely entwined with the
hugely popular ghost stories of the period. The anecdotes of
parasomnias seem to mimic tales of the supernatural, but ghost
stories are equally reminiscent of these real experiences. And if
we can apply a scientific eye to the cases presented by the Society
for Psychical Research, then surely we can do the same thing to
works of fiction.

☆　☆　☆

Patrick Lafcadio Hearn (1850–1904) was a Greek–Irish writer
who devoted much of his life to capturing the stories, folklore
and culture of late-nineteenth-century Japan. While there are
some aspects of Hearn's writing that rather romanticise and
exoticise Japanese culture, other parts of his work are important
for their preservation of ancient stories and tradition. In particular, he made Japanese stories accessible to English-language
readers. *Oriental Ghost Stories* (1904), for example, is a collection
of strange, creepy, and comedic supernatural tales he encountered during his life in Japan.

Ghost stories often focus on the bed and sleep, which makes
some of them worth analysing from the point of view of parasomnias rather than the supernatural. Japan's ghost stories are no
different. Within Hearn's collection is a story called 'Yuki-Onna'
(meaning 'Snow Woman'). It follows two woodcutters: Mosaku,
an old man, and his apprentice Minokuchi, aged eighteen. One
day, while heading home, the two men found themselves overtaken by a terrible snowstorm and needed to find shelter as

quickly as possible. They came across a seemingly abandoned ferryman's hut, and went inside to hide away from the blizzard. Mosaku fell asleep soon after lying down, but Minokuchi lay awake listening to the wind and the snow against the shabby, cold hut. Eventually, though, he fell asleep too. Hearn then writes:

He was awakened by a showering of snow in his face. The door of the hut had been forced open; and, by the snow-light (*yuki-akari*), he saw a woman in the room – a woman all in white. She was bending above Mosaku, and blowing her breath upon him – and her breath was like a bright white smoke. Almost in the same moment she turned to Minokuchi, and stooped over him. He tried to cry out, but found he could not utter any sound. The white woman bent down over him, lower and lower, until her face almost touched him; and he saw that she was very beautiful – though her eyes made him afraid. For a little time she continued to look at him – then she smiled, and whispered: 'I intend to treat you like the other man. But I cannot help feeling some pity for you – because you are so young ... You are a pretty boy, Minokuchi; and I will not hurt you now. But, if you ever tell anybody – even your own mother – about what you have seen this night, I shall know it; and then I will kill you ... Remember what I say!'

With these words, she turned from him, and passed through the doorway. Then he found himself able to move; and he sprang up, and looked out, but the woman was nowhere to be seen; and the snow was driving furiously into the hut.[12]

Minokuchi checked on his old master, Mosaku, and found him dead and cold to the touch. He was deeply affected by what he had seen and experienced, and it took him a long time to recover.

A year later, though, Minokuchi returned to his profession. One day, he met a beautiful young woman called O-Yuki. They soon got married, and had ten children. Seeing his wife sewing by the light of a paper lamp, Minokuchi reminisced about the ghostly woman he had seen when he was eighteen, and told his wife about the encounter. Naturally, O-Yuki turned out to *be* the ghost, and gave Minokuchi a dire warning that if their children ever had cause to complain about their father, she would kill him. With that, she disappeared for ever.

What is particularly interesting about this story is the way it must have reminded Hearn of his own childhood. Published posthumously in 1905, *Shadowings* is a book of essays, auto-biographical anecdotes, and miscellaneous writing. One of the pieces in this book is called 'Nightmare-Touch', in which Hearn describes his traumatic experiences of a strange kind of sleep paralysis.

In this essay, he writes about his childhood fear of the dark, but the *way* he writes feels quite child-like in itself. The old terrors seem to come back to him, and he almost pleads with the reader to take him seriously where the adults in his life had not – and made his life miserable because of it. Perhaps it's because my own sleep is similarly troubled, but I feel an overwhelming sense of sympathy – even anger – for the young boy in Hearn.

He prefaces his anecdotes by saying that as far back as he can remember, he had always experienced 'ugly dreams' which routinely manifested as hallucinations and other parasomnias.[13] He often complained of his sleep to the adults in the house, but was met with an exceptionally cruel lack of interest. Sleeping in what was called the Child's Room, he was not allowed a night light. In this household, a fear of the dark was a sign of weakness that must be stamped out: Hearn was told that it would not be tolerated and to get over it.

Hearn was clearly still adversely affected by this time in his life when he wrote: "'Nothing will hurt you,' – this was the merciless answer to all my pleadings not to be left alone at night. But the haunters *did* hurt me. Only – they would wait until after I had fallen asleep, and so into their power, – for they possessed occult means of preventing me from rising or moving or crying out.'

The episodes themselves are terrifying to read, let alone experience first-hand. They're likely sleep paralysis, but of a very repetitive and unusual sort. Each encounter with the shadowy figures that relentlessly tormented him begins with a creeping sense of dread. He knew what was coming, every time.

Happy voices I could hear in the next room; – I could see light through the transom over the door that I had vainly endeavoured to reach; – I knew that one loud cry would save me. But not even by the most frantic effort could I raise my voice above a whisper ... And all this signified only that the Nameless was coming, – was nearing, – was mounting the stairs. I could hear the step, – booming like the sound of a muffled drum, – and I wondered why nobody else heard it. A long, long time the haunter would take to come, – malevolently pausing after each ghastly footfall. Then, without a creak, the bolted door would open, – slowly, slowly, – and the thing would enter, gibbering soundlessly, – and put out hands, – and clutch me, – and toss me to the black ceiling, – and catch me descending to toss me up again, and again, and again ... In those moments the feeling was not fear: fear itself had been torpified by the first seizure. It was a sensation that has no name in the language of the living. For every touch brought a shock of something infinitely worse than pain, – something that thrilled into the innermost secret being of me, – a sort of abominable electricity, discovering unimagined capacities of suffering in totally unfamiliar regions of sentiency ...

The worst thing about sleep paralysis is how extraordinarily real it all feels. A hypnopompic hallucination is just an image; it might look real, but it quickly dissipates. With sleep paralysis, you *feel* what you see. If there's a shadowy figure above me, I can feel each of their fingers gripping my shoulders and their bony knees pressing into my stomach. I can feel their hot breath on my face. If someone only experienced it once in their life and never again, especially in an unfamiliar bedroom, it would be understandable if they misinterpreted it as supernatural in origin.

If you delve deep enough into TripAdvisor hotel reviews, you can find people to whom this has happened. A review from 2009 of The Wellington Hotel, Cornwall, bears the somewhat ironic title: 'DON'T STAY HERE ... IT'S A NIGHTMARE!!!!!'[14] Upon checking in to the hotel, the reviewer discovered a pamphlet describing the supposed supernatural phenomena that occurred there. It had, they write, even been visited by the (incredibly dubious) ghost-hunting television show *Most Haunted*. Already, then, the reviewer was anxious about encountering the ghosts that were rumoured to linger in the hotel, and in their room in particular.

The reviewer says that they were so nervous to be in the dark that they switched on the television and left it at a low volume. The reviewer slept through the night and woke up a little too early to get dressed for breakfast. They decided to lie in bed watching the television. Suddenly, they felt overwhelmed with dread, and said to themselves, 'It's here.' Someone seemed to be walking towards them where they lay prone in bed. A cold rush of air passed over them, followed by a 'total paralysis of my body ... I couldn't move I was frozen.'

The reviewer doesn't describe a figure beyond the feeling that someone was with them. The paralysis lasted for around thirty seconds, and then they found they could move again. The last part of the review describes the receptionist seemingly entertaining (but not in a particularly sensitive way) the reviewer's idea that they had encountered a ghost. There was a bit of an altercation, apparently, which led to the guest leaving a one-star review.

It may be that the ghost stories the reviewer had read before going to sleep contributed to the association of sleep paralysis and the supernatural. If this had happened in a new, corporate hotel in the middle of Manchester, would the reviewer have thought they had been visited by a ghost? Or would they even have had sleep paralysis at all? Clearly, the things the reviewer had read and been told about the hotel had already agitated them and may have contributed to disrupted sleep.

Over a century earlier, in *Phantasms of the Living*, Gurney, Myers and Podmore explained this phenomenon as 'expectancy'. If you convince yourself you're going to see a ghost, then you'll probably have a spooky nightmare or hallucination. They present an anecdote from a barrister in 1885 that has a strong parallel to the TripAdvisor review. The barrister was staying at a hotel with his friend K., a fellow lawyer. He thought that a door connected his room to K.'s, and when he told him about it, K. responded that he would come in during the night and frighten him. What a lad. But then the barrister opened the door and discovered that it wasn't actually connected to K.'s room, and went to bed without giving it another thought. He then writes:

> I must have been asleep some hours, when I woke up with a sensation that someone was close to my bed, and feeling about the other side of the chintz curtain at the head of the bed. I could hear the rustling and crackling of the curtain close to my face.

I've just realised how very lucky I am to live in an era where bed curtains are no longer part of the standard hotel experience. The barrister then describes a clear experience of sleep paralysis:

> I felt perfectly unable to move, or protect myself – not through any fear, but from a want of power of movement. After a few seconds this powerlessness went off, and I sprang out of bed, and saw the figure of my friend K. retreating towards the foot of the bed. He kept his face averted, his head a little bent, but I could see the wire and one of the glasses of his spectacles as he turned from me; he was dressed in his night-shirt. And what made me believe in the reality of the appearance was the 'solidity' of the white nightdress, and the light on the spectacles. [...] I grasped at my friend with both

hands and supposed I had missed him as my hands
met in the grasp. I attempted again to grasp him,
when he disappeared as if through the floor under the
washing-stand.

Sadly, we don't get K.'s reaction at the breakfast table when the
barrister tells him about this, but the anecdote does conclude
with a note from K. saying he doesn't have a history of sleepwalking (or vanishing through floorboards). Even though the
barrister knew K., the anecdote is still very creepy, especially
since he was in an unfamiliar bed. He brushes it off as a fascinating hallucination. If the barrister had expected to see a ghost,
though, and the figure wasn't someone he recognised, I wonder
how he would have told this story. Would he have found it to
be a strange and funny little anecdote, or would he have reacted
in the same way as the TripAdvisor reviewer, telling his friends
he had seen a ghost?

☆ ☆ ☆

Overall, what we see during sleep paralysis has changed significantly as our cultural depictions of monsters have shifted. No
one in the eighteenth century was seeing little grey aliens or
a chainsaw-wielding murderer in their sleep, and yet this is a
prevalent trope of twenty-first-century sleep paralysis. What
we consume in terms of images and fiction and culture shapes
what our imagination conjures up in the middle of the night.
Sometimes, when I ill-advisedly watch a scary film, I hope I
don't see its monster clambering up my bed at night. After sitting through *The Exorcist* for the first time, I barely slept at all

for fear that I might have sleep paralysis and get hallucinatory pea soup splattered on my face.

Sleep paralysis, in fact, is thought to be the cause of many reports of alien abduction. As quite a few of the anecdotes show, there's a peculiar sensation of weightlessness at the end of an episode. You feel as though you weigh the same as an elephant, and then suddenly the burden is lifted and it's like you're floating. In one of my own experiences described earlier, I felt myself rise up and then plunge over the side of my bed, only to wake with a jolt in my usual position, having not moved at all. This feeling, if the hallucination while paralysed was one of aliens, could be interpreted as being beamed back to Earth via a UFO's telekinetic rays.

Fortunately, inasmuch as you can be fortunate when you experience sleep paralysis, I've never hallucinated an alien abduction during an episode. I think that might just finish me off. But as a few teams of sleep researchers have found, it is now quite common for people to convince themselves of alien abduction after an attack of the *mara*. Just as the cultural anxiety of the supernatural in the seventeenth century led to a panic about witches, our modern monsters are the stuff of gory horror movies and the infinite unknowns of space exploration.

An investigation from 2005 by Richard J. McNally and Susan A. Clancy looked specifically at whether the anecdotes of those who believed they had been abducted by aliens could be reasonably explained by sleep paralysis. They found that eight of their participants had a common experience of seeking the help of a hypnotist to 'recover' memories of being abducted by aliens, and that these memories turned out to be highly sexual and invasive in nature.[15]

The actual reports of the 'abduction', however, are fairly mundane. They take place at night, in the sleeper's dark bedroom, and involve the usual symptoms of paralysis – which isn't just an inability to move, but a peculiar, heavy, charged feeling – and visual hallucinations of figures. Here's an example from McNally and Clancy's article:

> Another female abductee was lying on her back when she woke up in the middle of the night. She was completely paralyzed, and felt electrical vibrations throughout her body. She was sweating, struggling to breathe, and felt her heart pounding in terror. When she opened her eyes, she saw an insectlike alien being on top of her bed.

Through investigating the participants' mental health, the researchers didn't find evidence of any severe conditions such as schizophrenia. They hypothesised that these people may have experienced sexual abuse, perhaps in early childhood and since forgotten or repressed, but the results were inconclusive. What they did find, though, was that those who believed they had been abducted by aliens had more of an interest and active belief in frequent alien contact and Roswell-style conspiracy theories.

Parasomnias always involve a sleeper's fearful, confused or aggressive response to something only they can see. One of the differences, though, is whether the episode is remembered in the morning. I can't tell whether I'm lucky or unlucky to have parasomnias where I'm at least somewhat aware of myself and what's going on. I'm more inclined to say it's a good thing; I don't sleepwalk as often these days, but I remember the uncanny feeling of waking up to some sort of minor destruction and having no recollection of doing it. Now, even if the object itself is fuzzy by the morning, I always know that *something* happened in the night. And more often than not, I wake myself up in the middle of doing something strange – my own movements seem to snap me out of it fairly quickly.

But there's a parasomnia where forgetfulness is one of the key characteristics: night terrors. It's somewhere between sleepwalking and hypnopompic hallucinations – a person gets up in the night, most often in a state of absolute distress, and crashes around in an attempt to flee from some danger or disaster. There's often quite a lot of screaming involved, too. In the next chapter, I'll explore this phenomenon, from its early understanding as something that afflicted only young children, to the emergence of night terrors as a post-traumatic symptom in First World War soldiers.

Chapter 5

Night terrors

On Sunday 26 April 1908, members of America's own branch of the Society for Psychical Research sat around a table in the home of Mr and Mrs Cowper to commune with any nearby spirits. They used the method of the 'planchette' – a teardrop-shaped piece of wood that holds a pencil. The sitters gently touch the wood, lending their energy to the visiting ghost, and the planchette 'writes' at the behest of the dead. Their results were recorded in the Society's journal, and, as the editor describes in a preface, they 'largely explain themselves'. After a long night of vague and nonsensical messages from the afterlife, the group were tired and wanted to cut to the chase. Mr Cowper put his hand back on the planchette to give it one last go. The report reads as follows, with the sitters' questions written in brackets:

What do you want?
(We want to know who you are?)
Rita, Rita – We are all in hell, hell, hell, Hell is full.
We all have our hell in ourselves.

(What is the matter with Rita?)

Too many men for my husband.

(Are there no influences above you then that can help you?)

They never did on earth.

(Don't you know there are influences that can help you now?)

It will take a long time to wipe my child's blood from my hands.

(Can we help you?)

Help! Hell! You starve me and kill my child but I will get light.

(Have you anything to say to us?)

Don't believe the priest. He is the one – he lies.

By this time the four sitters were quite worked up. [Mr Cowper], who is a singularly robust man, was very pale and confessed to cold chills going up and down his spinal column. A normal, healthy child who was soundly sleeping in a room above woke up screaming loudly – we did not inquire if 'the cat's in the water butt,' but adjourned.[1]

For the group, the sudden sound of a screaming child piercing the night was enough to make them abandon their spooky conversation. As we've seen in previous chapters, the expectation of a ghost can be enough to wreak havoc on our imaginations. After the above quote finishes, the report offers no further description or analysis of the events; the group wants us to believe, as they clearly did, that the startling reaction from the sleeping child upstairs is related to the threatening messages being relayed through the planchette. Somehow, the spirit moving the pencil reached out its influence to the child upstairs at the exact moment when the sinister tone reached its peak. A dramatic climax to the evening. It makes for a chilling tale, but to read this from a sceptical perspective, and through the lens of sleep disorders, the report has a different interpretation.

The child, we can suggest, was experiencing a parasomnia known as the night terror. These have distinct characteristics: they seem to affect children most commonly, and involve the sleeper bolting out of bed in a state of abject fear. Those who suffer with night terrors run from unseen disasters and threatening situations, letting out a scream so genuine and loud that it tears through the stillness of the night. And when they wake up, they can't remember a thing. We don't learn from the report what happened to the child after the scream, but it's highly likely they easily drifted off back to sleep after the episode while the adults were reluctant to dim their bedroom lights. Often, the night terror is much more upsetting for those who witness its effects than it is for the sleeper.

☆　☆　☆

In her pioneering text, *Sleep: Its Physiology, Pathology, Hygiene, and Psychology* (1897), Russian physician Marie de Manacéïne describes night terrors as follows:

> It is probable that various distinct phenomena are commonly included under the name of nightmare. Thus the severe form called *pavor nocturnus*, or night terrors, and occurring only in early life, is a distinct affection.

It appears only between the second and eighth year; there is always a neurotic family history, and convulsions have been a frequent precursor. At the same time there may be no other sign of ill health. In night-terrors the onset is marked by a sharp cry; the child sees some object which inspires him with terror, he springs from his bed, crouches in a corner and protests vociferously. He recognises no one, and in the morning has no recollection of what has happened. The same vision is likely to reappear in future attacks; and it is held by some that this affection is allied to epilepsy.[2]

Night terrors, like many other parasomnias, were misunderstood for quite a long time. In particular, they were considered to be a form of epilepsy in the early nineteenth century. Epilepsy itself was often confused with several other, separate conditions, and was a term sometimes used to describe any sort of sudden change in a person – not just seizures but passing confusion, dizziness, lethargy or memory loss. One such example can be found in the 1870 volume of the London periodical *The Medical Times and Gazette*. A paper submitted by James Russell, physician at the general hospital in Birmingham, offers some examples of night terrors that he associates with epilepsy, calling them episodes of 'epileptic delirium'.[3] He does, however, note the association between poor sleep and the triggering of epileptic fits, so – with the knowledge available at the time – it would have made sense to see night terrors as another symptom of the condition.

The confusion between night terrors and epilepsy aside, the examples Russell gives are wild. I wish I could find out more about them, as Russell is sadly quite brief in his anecdotes, which surely have a much more detailed story behind them. Here's what he describes:

> Now in epilepsy the account I have received respecting some patients as to what has occurred in their dreams, offers a very striking resemblance to the description given of the milder form of delirium from which others have suffered. The patients talk, 'moither', shout, cry, 'ramble' in their sleep. They wake in terror, with eyes glistening, heart palpitating, a wild expression of face, and in a profuse perspiration. Occasionally they see spectres. In some cases the acts of the dreamer are of a more special character. A boy always seemed in trouble; he was constantly trying to save from drowning his mother and his younger brother, and always selected these two members of his family as the subject of his dreams. His mother had for a long time been obliged to sit by him twice or thrice a week, and sometimes for several nights in succession. A child awoke screaming, threw up the window and leapt through; she looked greatly terrified, and 'her screams were fearful'. A girl started up in bed declaring she saw men getting in at the window, her eyes being widely open, and she remained in this condition for two or three hours. A woman dreamed that her child was not her own, and in her sleep went down stairs, hoping to find some one to take charge of it; she then returned to her own room, thinking how foolish it was to keep the child; she opened the window, and was 'considering' about throwing it out, when, luckily, some one entered.

Night terrors are most often described and studied in terms of children's health, but they can occasionally affect adults, too. And, as with several of the parasomnias we've seen, they can either be a precursor to illness or manifest without any known cause.

A similar parasomnia to night terrors is REM behaviour disorder (RBD). I mentioned this briefly in the chapter on sleepwalking, but it seems appropriate to discuss it further here. When we dream, our brains still send signals to our muscles to act out whatever it is we're doing in our dream. To stop us from causing harm to ourselves and others, our bodies become paralysed. Where sleep paralysis is the phenomenon of waking up while still in that paralysed state, RBD occurs when the sleeper is not paralysed, and so their movements in bed correspond to what's going on in their dream. At this point, you're probably thinking of a recent scary or violent dream you had, and wondering in horror what might have happened if you *actually* performed those movements of self-defence or aggression. For those who suffer with RBD, this is a very real concern.

The pattern of behaviour associated with RBD is quite similar to night terrors and sleepwalking. They all involve a sleeper performing complex actions, having conversations, and acting out some sort of strange or distressing situation that only they can see. All three parasomnias also feature forgetfulness – the sleeper has no idea what they got up to in the night unless they were recorded or a co-sleeper informed them.

But there are some subtle yet fascinating differences between them. A 2013 study by Ginevra Uguccioni and others sought to examine sleepwalking, night terrors and RBD to identify and better understand their separate characteristics.[4] In particular, they focused on dream content – finding a way to compare what sleepers dreamt about to what they did while having an episode of RBD or night terror. Because of their shared characteristics, Uguccioni grouped together night terrors and sleepwalking, in contrast to RBD.

While most dreams associated with their parasomnia were forgotten by the subject, the team found that the vast majority of participants could remember at least one instance in which what they acted out in the night reflected the dream they had.

One of the biggest contrasts between RBD and night terrors was the level of aggression exhibited by the sleeper. Those who experienced night terrors and sleepwalking seemed to experience 'misfortunes' that made them vulnerable, desperate to flee or to protect themselves. These included examples such as earthquakes, losing precious items, tragedy befalling a loved one. In nearly every case, the sleeper was a powerless victim, very much enacting a 'flight' response. Those who experienced RBD, however, were in 'fight' mode. They still recalled a dangerous situation – a burglar, a predator, a bar brawl – but a red mist seems to have descended along with the delusion. Rather than run away or cower like the sleepwalkers or sufferers of night terrors, the sleepers with RBD turned violent and faced the danger head-on, often lashing out, shouting, and unfortunately causing damage and injury to themselves or their family.

A curious case appears in the 1829 *Transactions of the Medico-Chirurgical Society of Edinburgh*. The Society was established in 1821 by Dr Andrew Duncan, with the objective of encouraging discussion and publication among medical practitioners in the city. Their *Transactions* collected letters and strange case studies from all around the world, and the case in question comes from A.H. Renton in Funchal, Madeira. He writes of Frederick Blandy, a five-year-old boy. On the day Frederick's illness started, he had been playing with his friend Anne, who had then developed some peculiar symptoms of lethargy and disorientation. Later, Frederick also started to behave oddly, but in a much more violent manner. His symptoms, moreover, largely mimicked those of night terrors. Frederick had a moment of zooming all over the place, not unusual for a young child. He then fell asleep, also not unusual for a young child. Renton describes his sleep as follows:

> Out of this [sleep], however, the boy suddenly awoke, screaming most violently, and in a state of such ungovernable delirium, that, in spite of the utmost efforts of his father to restrain him, he repeatedly dashed his head against such objects as were nearest to him, and bruised himself severely.[5]

As distressing as this sounds, it does seem like a typical episode of night terrors. But having already been called to look at the case of Anne, Renton wondered if the two children's illnesses were related. He thought that they both seemed intoxicated, and wondered if they had ingested something poisonous.

Poor Frederick. Out came the emetics used to induce vomiting. When they didn't work, Renton opted for a stomach-pump, swiftly followed by a 'stimulating enema', followed by frequent doses of castor oil – a laxative. Renton was going to get it out of Frederick, whatever it took.

During the assault on Frederick's digestive system, up came some seeds which a friend of Renton's later identified as belonging to *Datura arborea*, the angel's trumpet tree. These are incredibly poisonous, and can lead to various psychological effects such as hallucinations, delirium, and psychosis. Potent stuff for a five-year-old. The symptoms begin quickly, too – between half an hour to an hour after ingestion. Renton notes that nearly an hour had elapsed between Frederick eating the seeds and the appearance of symptoms. Once Renton was positive that nothing harmful remained in Frederick's stomach, he let the boy recover. Frederick soon perked up, and the following day Renton reported him 'quite well'.

Renton, in his closing remarks, seems rather shaken by the proceedings. He confesses that he didn't know what the seeds were, and even so, argues that the tree produces seeds so rarely that he would never have thought it possible to be poisoned by them. He offers his essay as a warning to fellow practitioners.

We've already seen a few examples of the link between strange sleep and illness, how one can lead to another and how their symptoms can overlap, but this anecdote is perhaps the most revealing. If Anne hadn't also displayed similar behaviour, would Renton have thought that the two children had eaten something poisonous? Would he have concluded that Frederick was having a particularly bad case of night terrors?

On the other side, it emphasises how similar parasomnias can be to the effects of mind-altering drugs, poisons, and psychoses. It is no wonder that the troubled sleeper in literature is often connected with madness or substance abuse, as we saw in the case of the laudanum-addled Franklin Blake in Wilkie Collins' *The Moonstone*.

Renton's anecdote sticks out for me because of the caring tone with which he writes, but there are dozens of examples where this isn't the case. The Victorian era wasn't particularly well-known for its kindness and sympathy towards children, and many of the presented case studies of parasomnias seem to lack Renton's concern. Perhaps this is because Renton's case turned out to be severe poisoning and not night terrors in their own right. Elsewhere, anecdotes remind me of Mr Gradgrind in Charles Dickens' *Hard Times*, forever reproaching his children for fanciful thinking and imagination.

One example from 1899 is particularly complex in its approach to this parasomnia. In his essay, 'On Night Terrors, Symptomatic and Idiopathic, with Associated Disorders in Children', Dr Leonard Guthrie presents a number of anecdotes, many from his experience as a consultant at Paddington children's hospital.[6] He can't seem to decide what night terrors are; as we've already seen, it was a condition often confused as a symptom of epilepsy, and Guthrie perpetuates the misunderstanding here, but he also flits between treating the cases seriously and presenting them as an amusing story. Sometimes, he seems to dismiss the child's distress entirely, and at other times in the essay he sympathetically compares cases to memories of his own troubled childhood sleep. Perhaps it was the culture and general attitude to children that makes Guthrie so undecided: he *wants* to be sympathetic, as seen in the use of his own anecdotes, but at the same time he doesn't want to appear to champion a child's well-being over cold, hard scientific fact.

'Indeed,' he says, 'I can recognise no distinctions between night terrors and nightmare.' The reason why night terrors in children involve these disturbing fits of screaming, Guthrie argues, is because children are generally scared of everything and apt to scream at frightening images or ideas. He mentions a hallucination he recently had while attempting to sleep off a fever; he saw a grey man sink into the floor, and 'should have yelled with terror at the sight', but he was a man of medicine, of course, and not 'a baby', and therefore 'watched the apparition with much interest'. Slight bending of the truth, there, I suspect.

He does, however, include some anecdotes which are suitably creepy. As my family often found when I was ambling about the house at night, there is nothing quite as chilling as the glazed expression or strange speech of a sleepwalking child. My episodes of sleepwalking were all rather sedate – still creepy, but at least I was quiet. When adults watch a child have a night terror, they find themselves being told of a mortifying danger that only the child can see. That must be pretty horrible to experience.

Most of the anecdotes are taken from child-patients at hospitals, and Guthrie demonstrates a relationship between night terrors and illness. These illnesses seem to range from head lice to mal-developed bones, but nonetheless foreshadow later work investigating this particular parasomnia as a symptom or precursor to disease. It calls to mind the declining health of Mina and Lucy in *Dracula*, and how their troubled sleep coincided with the vampire's attacks. In one of the anecdotes, Guthrie describes a little boy, aged eight, who had been admitted to Paddington children's hospital with an abscess. He was labouring under a persistent fever, which seems to have caused a prolonged night terror and delusion.

> On the night before I saw him he awoke at 9.30 screaming, 'Robbers! Murderers!' He hid his head under the bed-clothes, and, when uncovered, bit and tore at every one who approached. He recognised no one, but listened intently to the slightest sound, fancying that robbers

were coming to murder him. When I saw him the next day he was still full of the same delusions. He insisted that the whole of the hospital staff had been murdered, and that his attendants were burglars dressed up in nurses' clothes. He refused food on the ground that it was poisoned, and spat in all directions for several hours at a time. […] He was alternately noisy and dull, muttering 'thunder and lightning' to himself. (There had been a thunderstorm on the day that his attack began.) The condition of mania, with delusions, lasted for three days, and then gradually subsided.

Sometimes, particularly in the nineteenth century, night terrors were seen as congenital rather than something that might appear spontaneously. This anecdote is a good example of how night terrors, or attacks of delusion that mimic the parasomnia, can be isolated incidents caused by illness or trauma.

He also, to my great amusement, offers one possible explanation for a child's night terrors: maths. I'm sure we can all agree that our first foray into fractions was a bit of a nightmare, but Guthrie seems adamant that thinking about arithmetic when drifting off to sleep is likely to make a child wake up screaming.

☆ ☆ ☆

There's a famous scene at the beginning of Charlotte Brontë's *Jane Eyre* that suggests the experience of something like a night terror. The novel starts in Jane's unhappy childhood spent with her aunt, Mrs Reed, and obnoxious cousins. Jane is an outcast in the family, forever bullied and persecuted in typical Cinderella fashion. On one particular occasion, she finally stands up to her nasty cousin, John. When John goes to lash out at her, Jane fights back. But of course, when the adults arrive at the scene, John is purely the victim and Jane the mad aggressor. As punishment, she gets locked in the 'Red Room', a cold and disused bedroom where Mr Reed died nine years before.

In the first few hours of her confinement, it is still daylight in the Red Room and Jane sits, quietly seething, on a stool. She isn't particularly scared at this point, but already the thoughts of Mr Reed's death, as well as being confronted by her rather ghostly reflection in an old mirror, make her uneasy. 'Superstition was with me at that moment,' says Jane, 'but it was not yet her hour for complete victory.'[7] I think we've all felt this; perhaps in an old hotel room, or after reading or watching something spooky. You tell yourself you're being ridiculous, but the darker it gets, the more the prickling chill of fear seems to grow.

And then, 'Daylight began to forsake the red-room.' Jane starts to become more and more fearful, and loses herself in a fantasy of ghosts and supernatural revenge. It isn't clear whether Jane is awake or not, but she suddenly sees something strange in the room.

> Shaking my hair from my eyes, I lifted my head and tried to look boldly round the dark room: at this moment a light gleamed on the wall. Was it, I asked myself, a ray from the moon penetrating some aperture in the blind? No; moonlight was still, and this stirred; while I gazed, it glided up to the ceiling and quivered over my head. I can now conjecture readily that this streak of light was, in all likelihood, a gleam from a lantern, carried by some one

across the lawn: but then, prepared as my mind was for horror, shaken as my nerves were by agitation, I thought the swift-darting beam was a herald of some coming vision from another world. My heart beat thick, my head grew hot; a sound filled my ears, which I deemed the rushing of wings; something seemed near me; I was oppressed, suffocated: endurance broke down; I rushed to the door and shook the lock in desperate effort.

Then follows a great deal of commotion. Several adults rush in to see Jane, complaining that she was screaming in such a visceral, strange, urgent way that they were shaken by the noise. Mrs Reed comes, and cruelly dismisses Jane's fear as an attention-seeking act, and locks her back up in the room. Shortly afterwards, Jane describes herself as having a 'species of fit'. Brontë writes: 'The next thing I remember is, waking up with a feeling as if I had had a frightful night-mare, and seeing before me a terrible red glare, crossed with thick black bars. I heard voices, too, speaking with a hollow sound, and as if muffled by a rush of wind or water; agitation, uncertainty, and an all-predominating sense of terror confused my faculties.'

Jane finds herself being attended by the family physician, and surrounded by a number of adults who had treated her so unkindly and now look at her with grave concern. She soon recovers, although she never forgets the experience, and carries it with her for the rest of her life.

While this episode isn't explicitly described as a night terror, it shares a lot of features that suggest Charlotte Brontë had experienced or known someone who suffered with these attacks. It's important to include, though, as it clearly demonstrates the attitudes that adults can sometimes have towards children who have sleep problems. Jane's terror is dismissed at first, just as young Lafcadio Hearn's fears were brushed aside as we saw in the previous chapter, and it is only when the symptoms are physical, taking the form of a kind of fit, that a physician is brought to examine her. It might not be one of the biggest themes or messages of *Jane Eyre*, but it's still crucial: take children's night-time fears seriously. It feels real to them. A study conducted in 2001, for example, found discrepancies in interviews with parents about their children's night-time fears versus how the children themselves described them. Peter Muris and his team showed 176 children in the Netherlands a short picture-book that told the story of a child becoming fearful after their mother turns off their bedroom light and leaves them alone in the dark. The researchers then asked the children a series of questions about the frequency, severity, and content of their fears. The parents were then asked the same questions about their children. Over 73% of the children reported being afraid at bedtime; only 34% of parents agreed.[8] While Muris and his team don't speculate about *why* parents don't know the extent of their children's night-time fears, the report does propose that it is far more helpful to listen to children above their parents when addressing sleep problems.

☆ ☆ ☆

One of the most important moments in the study and understanding of night terrors was the aftermath of the First World War. The physical injuries sustained by soldiers were no longer seen as the only wounds caused by conflict. Serious study was beginning to take place to assess and treat the psychiatric damage with which soldiers and other military personnel were suffering. The umbrella term 'shell shock' was used to describe a range of symptoms that affected veterans' mental health, including nervousness, mood changes, and a variety of sleep disorders.

In 1918, the year the war ended, Canadian psychiatrist and co-founder of the American Psychoanalytic Association, John T. MacCurdy, published an important survey into these post-traumatic symptoms. He rejects the term 'shell shock', opting to give the symptoms a more serious name, which he also uses as the title of the book: *War Neuroses*. Observing and participating in the medical treatment of soldiers during the war, MacCurdy noticed that discussions and developments in medicine were almost wholly focused on physical and easily treatable ailments. Psychological wounds, he says, were 'met with indifference on the part of the bulk of the profession.'[9] His book, then, sought to outline the array of psychological symptoms he had witnessed in soldiers, demonstrate the severity of these conditions through detailed case studies, and offer possible treatment.

What MacCurdy notices most is the prevalence of night terrors and other sleep disorders that emerged after soldiers had spent time at the front. With each case study, MacCurdy presents the patient's history of night terrors alongside their age and occupation within the military. Night terrors in childhood, he suggests, indicate a high propensity for the horrors of war to re-emerge through this parasomnia.

The first case study is a harrowing demonstration of the suffering and torment experienced by soldiers on the front line. It also shows how, rather than a balm to a wounded mind, sleep can refresh and regurgitate the hellish scenes experienced, and prolong the feeling of terror even in a safe environment. This is the story of Case 1.

'The patient was a man of 27,' MacCurdy writes, 'who had never been ill in his life.' Unlike some of the other case studies presented, Case 1 did not have a childhood history of night terrors and was considered to be in good mental health prior to enlisting. In 1915, he was in the firing line in France, and broke out in a 'cold sweat with fear' during his first experience of being close to exploding shells. This was soon accompanied by a change in mood: he began to develop depression and a peculiar sleepiness.

Case 1 then takes a sad turn. He becomes too ill to continue fighting, and is admitted to hospital where MacCurdy meets him. 'To keep himself in hand he began to drink,' says MacCurdy. This worsened his quality of sleep, and had perhaps the opposite effect of what the patient wanted in that he started to experience strange phenomena in his sleep. His hypnagogic hallucinations – those flashes of scenes and images we experience before sleep – were more pronounced than is usual. Every time he closed his eyes, he was back at the Somme, about to be showered with bombs from above. He would enter half-asleep delusions, believing he would have to resume his position on the front the next day. These symptoms would stop him from truly falling asleep, as he would snap awake in fear as soon as they began to manifest.

The patient began to suffer from night terrors during his hospital stay. MacCurdy writes: 'In them he was back on the Somme front and being shelled mercilessly. Shells would come closer and closer to him, finally one would land right on top of him and he would awake with a shriek of terror. After a long time he would go to sleep again, to be almost immediately reawakened with another of these dreams, the content being always the same and confined to fighting, in which he was invariably getting the worst of it.' This coincides with more modern research into the delusions experienced by people suffering with night terrors – namely, that they are in imminent, life-threatening danger from which they have to flee. Clearly, the front line of the trenches was febrile ground for such constant and deadly threats. It's no wonder night terrors became such a key symptom of post-traumatic stress suffered by war veterans.

In the morning, the patient would be 'absolutely played out' from the trauma of reliving his experiences in his sleep. Unfortunately, Case 1 only becomes more tragic. MacCurdy notes: 'Then came the news of the death of one of his best friends in France, which depressed him considerably. Shortly after this a concert was arranged at the hospital and he tried to sing, but failed. This experience made him much worse. The old dreams began to destroy his sleep with great regularity.' It isn't clear what happened to the patient afterwards; MacCurdy ends the anecdote there, without mentioning whether the man improved or not.

Another patient, Case 22, exhibited particularly violent night terrors. This man was only 23 years old when he was brought to the hospital for treatment. When he first displayed signs of trauma, he suffered from restless nights in which the horrors of the front were replayed to him. But unlike the man in Case 1, these evolved in content as time went on. He stopped seeing specific images of war – shells, the battlefield, bayonets lunging towards him – and instead experienced the overwhelming and disastrous scenarios so common to night terrors. For example, 'he would dream that the hospital was on fire, or that Zeppelins were going to come.' MacCurdy offers a particularly interesting anecdote: 'Once while sleeping on a balcony he dreamed that it collapsed but that he hung on to the edge with his fingers. He awoke screaming to the nurse to come and rescue him.'

For MacCurdy, night terrors were one of the most important indicators of trauma. But he writes with a sense of frustration, presenting a number of cases as a way of drawing attention to the severity of symptoms that he felt were overlooked by other medical practitioners. At the beginning of *War Neuroses*, he urges doctors to see psychological damage in the same light as physical wounds. However, even this view is problematic, as MacCurdy seems to consider emotional trauma as something which can be healed with as much success as an injury to the flesh or bones. On one hand, the cases in *War Neuroses* are all written with a sense of overwhelming sympathy and a need to help the patients MacCurdy encounters. But towards the end of the book he suggests that if psychological and physical wounds are held in the same regard, then treatment for traumatised soldiers can be perfected, and those soldiers can then resume their duties. The patient, he says, 'should be assured that because his disease is curable, he will, of course, have to return [to the battlefield] eventually.'

Despite MacCurdy's belief that the night terrors of soldiers were 'curable' in much the same way as a bullet wound or broken leg, his work was influential in understanding how parasomnias can occur as a result of trauma. This was particularly important for night terrors, which were thought to be present only in children. MacCurdy was at the forefront of showing how such conditions could re-emerge, or even appear for the first time in a person's life, because of the horrors they had experienced. He also demonstrated how varied and subjective were the wounds suffered by soldiers; the injuries sustained from war, he showed, were often far more complex than physical wounds.

☆ ☆ ☆

As with the other parasomnias already looked at, different cultures offer a multitude of explanations for night terrors. Common among them is a link to the supernatural. In south-west Nigeria, for example, the Yoruba community call the phenomenon *ogun oru,* meaning 'nocturnal warfare'. In their article investigating the subject, Lagos-based researchers of psychiatric medicine O.F. Aina and O.O. Famuyiwa surveyed a traditional Yoruba healer and three clergymen and found some variety in their belief of what *ogun oru* involves. Where two clergymen described it as a form of punishment inflicted on women by their 'spirit husbands', the healer and the other clergyman blamed the condition on being given food in a dream by a witch. The latter involves a folkloric theory that to dream of eating leads to being poisoned, an explanation for illness. It is described by Aina and Famuyiwa as having several characteristics: '(1) the person is attacked at night while asleep; (2) the illness is attributable to being poisoned by an enemy through eating in the dream, as revealed by a divination performed by a traditional healer; (3) the sufferer awakens and is unable to sleep again; (4) he or she behaves in an agitated and abnormal manner and may cry out like a goat.'[10]

Aina and Famuyiwa present several case studies of people within the Yoruba community who were afflicted with parasomnias. They show the modern clash of traditional and scientific intervention for sleep disorders. One of the cases, Miss IA, presents a particularly sad story.

Miss IA, a 34-year-old tailor, presented to the clinic with a 5-month history of intermittent disturbed behavior usually exhibited at night. During such nights, she was unable to sleep and shouted at the top of her voice, but during the day, she was socially withdrawn. Such episodes would last for one or two days and thereafter she would be symptom-free for two to four weeks before another episode. Some neighbors labeled her problem as *ogun oru*. Past history revealed that she had developed a night-time wandering behavior with destructiveness about six years previously and was reportedly treated by an herbalist.

Relatives firmly believed the illness was spiritual and probably arose from a family curse. When seen in the clinic, she was dressed in the white garments of members of the church from where she was brought. History from her sister revealed that the patient had been taken to the church for spiritual care under the supervision of a prophet about six weeks prior to presentation in the clinic. While in the church, she underwent rites meant to sever her ties to a spirit husband who was believed to be responsible for her having remained single until the age of 34, and also had deliverance sessions to relieve the probable family curse. Two red candles (made in the form of a small human) were tied back-to-back and suspended upside down. The name of the patient was invoked on one of the candles and the spirit husband invoked on the other. Prayers were recited for seven consecutive nights to turn the two against each other. Thereafter, the candles were lit and left to burn out.

It was believed that as the candles burnt out, so the relationship between the patient and spirit husband would be severed. The deliverance from curses involved prayers and fasting, as well as bathing with spiritual water.

When these interventions didn't provide much help to the woman, she was taken to hospital for treatment. Her test results came back normal until, sadly, she died some months later of typhoid fever.

Across Africa, as Aina and Famuyiwa illustrate, there are widespread beliefs in an immaterial realm closely linked to the realm we live in. In the Yoruba community specifically, night is perceived as a time when the veil separating the two realms is at its thinnest. Night is when spirits, witches, demons, vengeful ghosts of ancestors and other supernatural enemies can cross over to wreak havoc on sleeping mortals. And as we saw in the case above, the first course of action for those afflicted with troubled sleep is a spiritual, rather than medical, intervention.

☆ ☆ ☆

Night terrors are not something I have ever experienced, but my cousin, Olivia, has struggled with them for many years, seeking treatment at sleep clinics and making lifestyle changes in an attempt to stop them.

I talk to Olivia about sleep quite a lot – it's nice, in a way, to know someone in the family who experiences strange things in the night. We share anecdotes and worries, and have moments of wide-eyed surprise and relief when we realise that we're not alone in what happens to us.

But where I would compare my parasomnias to quiet, sinister thrillers, Olivia's night terrors are full-blown horror movies.

At a family gathering, one of my sisters and I were chatting with Olivia in a separate room. The conversation inevitably turned to sleep.

Olivia pulled out her phone. 'I've got an app that starts recording when I make a sound in the night. Do you want to hear some?'

'Absolutely.'

She looked back at the door, a grin growing on her face. She scrolled through her phone for a few seconds.

'This one,' she said, laughing. 'This was in a Travelodge.'

My sister and I waited as Olivia pressed play. There was a muffled sound, some crackling static, and then a loud, drawn-out, gut-sinking scream. It was unlike anything I'd heard before, certainly far more chilling than even the most enthusiastic movie-scream. In fact, whenever I watch someone scream in a film now, I think about just how flat and fake it sounds in comparison to Olivia's recording. This was a scream of true fear – a pure, instinctive reaction to something that genuinely threatened survival. You couldn't mimic a scream like that. Certainly not in a busy Travelodge.

'Here's another one,' Olivia said, delighted by our expressions of shock.

She played the recording. There was a quick succession of words – Olivia was accusing someone of something. We heard a rapid thud of footsteps, and then a loud bang and crash.

'I ran into a lamp.'

I've downloaded similar sound-recording apps a few times, but the same self-consciousness comes back when I try to record myself, and I can't fall asleep if it's recording. I know it would be just for me, that I wouldn't have to share it with anyone, but I think I'd rather not know what this 'other' me gets up to in the night. Besides, for things like hypnopompic hallucinations or sleep paralysis, I don't make any kind of verbal noise apart from a sharp gasp, perhaps. All you'd hear is a quick shuffle of bedclothes, and the sound of me sighing at my own ability to be drawn into the delusion.

For all that we were laughing at the clips of Olivia dashing about, smacking into walls, swearing and screaming, night terrors have had a serious impact on her well-being. She sometimes puts herself in active danger, or does something that has ongoing consequences. When in university, she put her foot through her bedroom window, smashing the glass and needing hospital treatment. The university were less than sympathetic, perhaps because they didn't understand what night terrors were, and demanded that Olivia paid for repairs. When she was doing her PhD and attending conferences, she would sometimes overhear fellow delegates discussing the blood-curdling scream they heard in the hotel that night.

She worked at a university in the north of England for a few years, and while there she went to her first sleep clinic. I've never been to a sleep clinic because my eventful nights are too unpredictable – I don't want to waste their time by having an appointment and being too self-conscious to sleep, or having a completely normal night. For Olivia, though, her night terrors are an unfortunately frequent part of her life. The staff at the clinic measured her brainwaves and gave her the official diagnosis: her regular nightly awakenings were, indeed, night terrors. They attempted to treat her with clonazepam, a medication used to alleviate seizures and movement disorders as well as sleep-related problems. It has been used for many years as a way of decreasing the severity of night terrors; in 1992, for example, American neurologist Mario Mendez successfully lessened the number of episodes suffered by a young man, whose night terrors began after an operation to remove a tumour from his brain stem.[11]

Unfortunately, the medication didn't work for Olivia. One night, while she was on clonazepam, she woke up to find herself by her open bedroom window, about to jump out into the river far below. After that, whenever she went on a work-related trip her boss made sure she only slept in rooms on the ground floor of buildings.

Then, a few years ago, Olivia was in a house-share in her new job in London. Sure enough, her housemates soon came to learn the extent of the problem. For one person in particular, it was too much. He gave her an ultimatum: sort them out or leave. This was a tough time for Olivia. Her night terrors worry her. When we talked about them, we found we shared the same sense of unease that there's a part of ourselves we don't know and can't trust.

She re-embarked on her mission to get to the bottom of her parasomnia, and to try to get it treated. She went to see a few neurologists, with varying degrees of success. Because of the risks of addiction and negative side-effects associated with benzodiaz-epines such as clonazepam, non-pharmaceutical therapies have been and continue to be developed as an alternative to potentially harmful medication. In 1988, for example, Bryan Lask, a consultant psychiatrist at Great Ormond Street children's hospital, devised a technique that involved having parents watch their children for signs that a night terror was about to occur (racing heart, sweating, twitching), and then wake the child before the attack could begin.[12] He found this to be successful with all nineteen children he studied. Cognitive behavioural therapy and hypnosis are also used to try to pinpoint an underlying psychological cause for the night terrors. With one neurologist, Olivia underwent hypnotherapy, which she told me had a little bit of a beneficial effect – certainly more than the clonazepam. At another specialist, she was given a course of melatonin, a hormone that controls the sleep cycle. This didn't work, either. The last neurologist Olivia saw helpfully told her she would grow out of it, despite the fact that Olivia was 33 years old. Otherwise, she was told there was not much that could be done.

I hope Olivia eventually finds a way to calm her night terrors. When she was giving me the details of her experience at the sleep clinics, she told me that one of the things that troubles her the most is the stigma attached to these kinds of conditions, particularly in terms of madness and the supernatural. But as we saw in the opening chapter, around 70% of us will experience a parasomnia in our lives. We need to talk more about our strange nights, and understand that they're far more common and normal than we think.

Night terrors in children are distressing, but they're often seen as a fairly normal and common part of development. Usually, they grow out of it. An interesting fact about Agatha Christie, the famous mid-twentieth-century crime novelist, was that she appears to have suffered from night terrors as a child. These terrors centred on a dream which involved a recurring figure she called 'The Gunman'. He appeared as an eighteenth-century Frenchman, with powdered hair in a ponytail, pale and piercing blue eyes, and carrying a musket. The dream would otherwise be mundane; a pleasant afternoon in the garden, or a dinner party, but then The Gunman would appear to terrorise little Agatha. It doesn't seem as though Agatha was afraid of the gun he carried, or even that he tried to shoot her – it was simply his presence that terrified her. As she writes in her autobiography, it was the fact that he represented 'someone *who ought not to be there.*'[13] His eyes were what scared her the most; when he stared at her with his cold gaze, there was a sense of finality – there was no escaping him once he had seen her. Then Agatha would wake up screaming, shouting The Gunman's name.

These dreams seemed to plague her most when she was four years old, which is a common age for night terrors experienced in childhood. But The Gunman stayed with her throughout her life, re-emerging in her work or at times of particular stress. In her later childhood, for example, she experienced numerous disasters and tragedies. Her father died when she was eleven years old, and subsequently her mother suffered a series of heart attacks. At night, Agatha would struggle to get to sleep, fearful that her mother was having another heart attack somewhere in the house, and that she would be dead by the time Agatha got up in the morning. While her dreams never manifested again as night terrors, The Gunman seems to have lingered in her mind, representing all that she feared and dreaded. She writes about him in her autobiography, and her relatively little-known novel, *Unfinished Portrait*, fixates on the dreams of its female protagonist.

This isn't the only link between night terrors and the world of crime fiction. Ellis Peters, pseudonym of Edith Pargeter, uses the parasomnia as the basis of one of the books in the classic

Cadfael series. Written between 1974 and 1994 (and adapted for television, starring Derek Jacobi), *Cadfael* follows its titular detective, a medieval monk in Shrewsbury, as he tries to solve the latest grisly murder. The eighth book in the series, *The Devil's Novice* (1983), sees a young arrival at the abbey, Meriet, who is mysteriously desperate to take his vows. After witnessing a fellow novice injure himself on a scythe, however, Meriet seems to overreact as though reliving a past trauma. Cadfael is curious. That night, Meriet's night terrors begin. Peters writes a rather chilling description:

> The scream came rendingly, shredding the darkness and the silence, as if two demoniac hands had torn apart by force the slumbers of all present here, and the very fabric of the night. It rose into the roof, and fluttered ululating against the beams of the ceiling, starting echoes wild as bats. There were words in it, but no distinguishable word, it gabbled and stormed like a malediction, broken by sobbing pauses to draw in breath.[14]

The monks (bar the very sensible Cadfael) give Meriet the nickname of 'the devil's novice', believing him to converse with Satan rather than with God. While Peters describes the symptoms of night terrors with notable accuracy – Meriet cannot recall the episodes in the morning, and doesn't remember any associating dreams – there is a sense that they are confused with several different conditions of sleep. These outbursts of Meriet's are consistently called 'nightmares', or even an 'incubus' which, as we've seen, is quite a different experience altogether. They are, though, undeniably night terrors. And while they lend a slightly spooky atmosphere to the book, as sleep disorders seem to do as a plot device in fiction, Peters demonstrates through Cadfael's wisdom and lack of superstition that the boy is struggling with the effects of trauma, not the influences of the devil.

The Middle Ages had numerous theories on troubled sleep and its causes, both natural and supernatural. Common to all, though, was the understanding that the sleeper was not to be blamed for their actions in sleep. This was particularly important in terms of religious culture; for example, what was called 'nocturnal pollution' – erotic dreams and ejaculation while asleep – needed to be rationalised as an involuntary and therefore not a sinful act, especially to save embarrassment among high-ranking or esteemed members of the Church. In the case of Meriet, then, it's unlikely that the monks would have cast such immediate suspicion on him.

This isn't to say Peters was entirely inaccurate in the superstitious overreaction of her monks in *The Devil's Novice*. An idea proliferated that Satan and his minions could infiltrate a sleeper's vulnerable mind; while the victim was innocent in what they did while under a demon's influence, the fact remained that they *were* being manipulated. Saint Albert the Great (c. 1200–80), a German friar and philosopher, for example, believed that all angelic creatures, whether good or bad, could control a sleeper's imagination.[15]

☆ ☆ ☆

Children's night terrors are difficult to treat – as we've seen, medication such as benzodiazepines are only used in extreme cases as a last resort – but an interesting option was proposed by a team of researchers in 2018. Sean D. Boyden and his team present a theory that night terrors are a kind of lingering evolutionary trait from the days of early human societies.[16] For safety and warmth, families and communities would sleep closely together – to be alone in the dark was to be very vulnerable, especially for a child. In modern society, though, young children are often given their own bedrooms and trained to sleep by themselves, away from the rest of the family. The hypothesis, then, is that night terrors emerge from a primitive fear of the vulnerability of sleeping alone in the dark. If families mimicked the old way of sleeping as a group, they ask, would the child's night terrors improve? Further work needs to be undertaken to prove whether this is the case, but it proposes an interesting re-evaluation of 'sleep-training' children.

Another member of Boyden's team, Philip T. Starks, brings a personal angle to the research paper. His own three-year-old son suffered with severe night terrors, experiencing 'four to seven a week for several months'. Starks' family tried everything in an effort to improve the son's sleep, including changing his diet, protecting him from frightening or threatening imagery, and keeping to a strict sleep schedule. Nothing worked. It was by chance and 'possibly due to exhaustion' that Starks decided to co-sleep with his son in the same bed. According to the article, the son's night terrors quickly improved and then disappeared altogether.

I find this interesting, even if it might not be practical for many households. What I consider to be my first memory is one of being afraid at night. I was standing up, clutching the bars of my cot, being very scared and not sure why. I remember my Dad bending over me, trying to soothe me. When I was very young, three or four years old, I used to be an absolute pain at night. I couldn't sleep on my own; I used to go into my parents' room, the corner of my pillow clutched in my little fist and trailing behind me, and plead to spend the rest of the night in their bed. For young children, night and darkness are terrifying. Even before the imagination has been populated with creepy clowns, ghosts and monsters, children know that there is danger in being alone in the dark. Maybe Boyden and his team are not far from the truth, in terms of night terrors being a kind of evolutionary separation anxiety.

☆   ☆   ☆

Night terrors are one of the more mysterious parasomnias. More so than hallucinations or sleep paralysis, there seems to be a significant split in terms of the causes of the phenomenon. On the one hand, they can have no particular underlying condition. They are simply something a person has on occasion, or, more commonly, a side-effect of a child's development in their early years. However, night terrors also seem to have a darker edge, which is that they can be a result of traumatic experiences, or a symptom or a precursor of a serious disease such as dementia.

In 1994, a team of psychiatrists in Bristol used paroxetine to treat an adult woman's night terrors successfully.[17] Paroxetine is a common antidepressant used for a range of mental health problems such as panic attacks, anxiety, and obsessive-compulsive disorder. In the study, the 46-year-old woman had a long history of sleep problems. She sounds a little like me: she sleepwalked as a child, then improved, but then developed a much more serious array of parasomnias following several years of stress in a turbulent marriage that ended in divorce. By the time she was engaged to a new partner, her night terrors had become so bad that it was affecting the relationship – she would have two or three episodes a night, every night. She had a regular bedtime and sleep schedule, but would wake up soon after falling asleep with a racing heart, sweating, shortness of breath and a feeling of intense fear. When the episode subsided, she would be confused and couldn't remember what had happened or what had made her feel so afraid. In the daytime, she was groggy and had difficulty concentrating.

The woman was extremely distressed, and began to drink heavily in order to knock her out at bedtime. She had tried a range of medical treatments before, such as diazepam, but wanted to be taken off it and reduced her dosage. The researchers at Bristol tried her with a combination of paroxetine and clonazepam, and found her night terrors improved immediately and dramatically. When they gradually stopped the dosage of clonazepam, they found that her night terrors didn't come back, leading them to believe that the paroxetine on its own worked enough to treat her nightly episodes. She stopped drinking alcohol, and after eight months of the trial had had the longest night-terror-free period for fifteen years.

Night terrors are perhaps one of the lesser-understood parasomnias. Perhaps it's because they aren't as 'romantic' as the others. If they're presented in fiction, it's as a symptom of PTSD, but even then as a rather mild form of the traumatised protagonist sitting bolt-upright in bed and screaming. They don't have the erotic undertones of sleep paralysis, nor the calm, away-with-the-fairies behaviour of the sleepwalker. They are frightening, messy, and loud; they don't make for good viewing. But that doesn't mean they are not worth talking about; if anything, there needs to be more representation of their effects and stories of lived experience. As we've seen, this could be especially important for children, whose night-time fears and troubled sleep might be difficult to communicate. As neuroscientists and psychologists continue to work to understand this distressing sleep disorder, we should also work to find ways to express night terrors.

Where night terrors have a relative lack of representation in stories and culture, there's one aspect of sleep that has been documented for thousands of years: dreams. This by-product of sleep has influenced the imagination more than any other parasomnia, and has been studied in every discipline and manifested in every art form. In the next chapter, we will explore some of the theories, studies, and artistic representations of the lives we live and the places we go when we're asleep.

Chapter 6

Narrating dreams

On 4 October 1939, Mrs G. Dean – a young woman from Portsmouth – wrote down her dream as part of a Mass Observation survey. Beginning in 1937, the Mass Observation project sought to document the everyday lives of the British public in the form of diaries or questionnaires. During the Second World War, it became a way for researchers to see the personal impact of news, propaganda and restrictions. In Mrs Dean's dream, the war is clearly on her mind:

> One fantastic scene I remember was a churchyard which suddenly became flooded with about 3 feet with a [thick] dark fluid, with masses of weeds and cords and wire-ends floating about. This dream took place the same night as I had seen photos of these gas-bags for young babies in the papers and was no doubt responsible for the ending of this dream.
>
> My own son, who figured in that ghastly dream, I wrote about a month or so ago, had been playing about

in this churchyard and was missing. We searched frantically and all the time this liquid was creeping up and
covering all the pathways. In desperation I started to
grope among the weeds and felt a long shape. I pulled it
up and there was my son as snug as a diver in his suit,
inside one of these gasbags.

This was the only dream I remember from beginning
to end. The others fade almost as soon as I awaken, but I
do know that the war is affecting my nightly escapades.[1]

It is one of hundreds of similar reports submitted to the social
research organisation during the conflict, in a special investigation on the content of people's dreams. What they were
particularly interested in was whether dreams, particularly
negative, anxiety-based dreams, were being influenced by the
proliferation of news bulletins and propaganda that painted a
grim picture of the war's progress.

The dreams are fascinating; each has its own stories and
characters, and offers intimate glimpses into the ordinary lives
and anxieties of the British public. Some are only apologetic
sketches a few sentences in length; others are long, detailed, ram-
bling narratives that seem to delight in the fact that someone is
interested in reading something so strange and private. Many of
the dreams involve the war. Images of violence, panic of hiding
from or being chased by the enemy, and the apocalyptic wail of
air raid sirens punctuate otherwise ordinary dreams of shopping,
walking in the park, or being unprepared for a school exam.
While some, like Mrs Dean, notice how the war is affecting their
sleep, some of the dreams in the collection are written without
particularly acknowledging the proliferation of war imagery.

In fact, the war becomes part of the fabric of their sleep, and some participants in the Mass Observation survey are more interested in other aspects of dreams.

Nancy Brown, a librarian from Bideford, submitted multiple dreams to the survey. Hers are quite short, but she is enthusiastic in her self-reflection. The explanatory notes she offers demonstrate how the frequency of war-themed dreams became part of the norm. One of the most interesting dreams from Nancy's collection was typed on 29 September 1939. She writes:

> An air-raid. I sheltered in an upstairs room with some children. They would press their noses against a [French] window. The windows were smashed in but the children were only slightly injured. I had to bind up their hands.
>
> NB Result I think of going to [the film version of] 'Wuthering Heights' on Saturday, and seeing Heathcliff deliberately putting his hands through the glass of his window and later having them bound up by Flora Robinson.

The movies feature a few times in Nancy Brown's dreams. She dreams of Stalin after watching a gangster film, for example. It's always the film itself that holds most significance in Nancy's mind. The war becomes something of a background prop.

In a report drawn up during the investigation, the Mass Observation group discuss whether the content and imagery of propaganda was to blame for the violent and fearful images in the dreams they received. In a section titled 'Application of the foregoing material to conduct of the country during war time', the writers suggest that a 'middle course should if possible be steered, by propaganda, between mixing of values – too much emphasis on the niceness of the Germans – and over-marshalling of aggression through too much emphasis on brutality of the enemy.'[2] They wondered if a change in tone would benefit the public; perhaps they could shift the content of the public's dreams from images of the enemy to scenes of British victory.

☆ ☆ ☆

We experience dreams during cyclical periods of REM-stage sleep that get progressively longer as we reach the end of our natural sleeping pattern. They are thought to be a way for our brains to sift through memories and experiences, embedding the things we learn or regurgitating the things we've seen or thought about during the day. They can be mundane or fantastical, snatches of images or fully-formed narratives, vivid or monochrome. We all dream multiple times a night, even if we don't remember them when we wake up.

The history of dreams is long and complex, with shifting attitudes and culturally specific ideas and interpretations. In the past, dreams have been seen as gifts from the gods, prophetic visions, demonic visitations, or simply the by-product of an overindulgence in meat and wine. More so than today, the dreams of antiquity were often taken as portents. Wars were waged, and statues were built or moved hundreds of miles, because of a supposedly divine dream. To have a god appear in a dream, and give the dreamer a message, was a sure sign of the dreamer's importance and status. On the other hand, interpreting dreams as prophetic has led to disastrous choices. In Robert Gray's *The Theory of Dreams* (1808), he relates an anecdote of a Welsh man who dreamt of riches buried beneath the head-stone of a holy well.

He travelled there, and when he plunged his hand in to retrieve his prize, he was bitten by an adder.[3] So the story goes, anyway.

Despite the emphasis on rationality and scientific inquiry placed on dreams in the Victorian era, the idea that dreams could be prophetic or telepathic had a bit of a revival. One of the most remarkable instances of this related to the frequent polar explorations being undertaken during the nineteenth century. Tales and images of the Arctic were widely printed and discussed, and it didn't take much for the explorers' chilling visions of isolation and extreme hardship to affect the minds of the reading public. Fridtjof Nansen's memoir of his polar expedition, *Farthest North* (1897), for example, was read by Sigmund Freud, who then dreamt of the Arctic. The Victorian public were fascinated by these alien landscapes; stories about the polar explorers often featured spooky visitations and strange spectres glimpsed on the snow – a phenomenon likely produced by extreme bodily and mental stress, but one that nevertheless appealed to an era obsessed with ghost stories and the Gothic.

But there is a particular type of dream associated with this period that is especially odd. When an expedition crew was deemed to be lost, the Victorian public mourned with their usual macabre gusto. Out of this mourning came the phenomenon in which a grieving widow or family received news of the crew's health, not from the crew themselves but from a fellow member of the public who had seen them alive and well in a dream.

This was especially common during the anxious and tragic period surrounding the loss of the Franklin expedition. It is a rather infamous disaster, but its impact on the British public is less discussed. Led by Captain Sir John Franklin in 1845, the expedition was formed of two ships: Franklin's HMS *Terror* and HMS *Erebus* captained by James Fitzjames. The aim was to investigate unmapped sections of the 'Northwest Passage', a treacherous sea route through the Arctic that linked the Atlantic and Pacific oceans and was considered vital for international trade at the time. If the expedition succeeded, then Britain would gain strength in its commercial power. But they never made it: both ships became locked in ice in what is now Nunavut, Canada. The crew, 129 men in total, stayed aboard the ships for over a year, during which time their number dramatically decreased – including the death of Franklin himself. Fitzjames and Franklin's second-in-command, Francis Crozier, as well as a handful of crew who had survived fates of lead poisoning, malnourishment, and exposure to Arctic temperatures, abandoned the ships in search of help. They were never seen again.

After two years without word from either ship, concern for the missing crew began to mount in Britain. From 1848, Captain Franklin's wife, Lady Jane Franklin, persuaded the government to fund numerous (and equally dangerous) rescue expeditions and handsome rewards for information. When the government refused to continue the search, declaring the crew legally dead in 1854, Lady Franklin put her own money towards a further expedition. Her grief was palpable and a popular topic of conversation. The mystery of Franklin and his crew was very much part of the Victorian imagination. More likely out of pity than trickery, Lady Franklin began to receive letters of hope from people, mostly women, who had received a vision of her husband through a dream.

Shane McCorristine, in his book *The Spectral Arctic*, describes this strange, somewhat sad phenomenon in detail. As quoted by McCorristine, Lady Franklin received the following letter from a correspondent in Southsea in 1850:

I saw in my dream two Air Bloon's a great distance off rising just like the moon. I said in my dream to myself [this is] Sir J. Frankland. I looket the second time as the Bloon's [rises?] on their journey looking beautiful an as I looket all in a moment one Banishet like a Pillar of Smoke. The second Bloon still going on its journey it gets to a place where I saw the inhabitants living People I saw in the my dream a Lady beautiful Dressed looking at them I said in my dream their is Lady Frankland but with this dream I saw nothing but snow as it fell amongst the inhabitants of these two Bloon's [*sic* throughout].[4]

While some of these accounts were directed straight to Lady Franklin herself, public interest in the expedition had grown so large that reports of psychic dreams were bypassing the family completely and going straight to the newspapers. In 1848, for example, the *Illustrated London News* describes a young woman from Bolton who, under mesmeric trance, claimed to 'visit [the] ships' in her sleep.[5] The tantalising mystery coincided with the popularity of clairvoyance and mesmerism, and it became something of a cultural phenomenon.

McCorristine demonstrates that 'it is clear that the [Franklin] loss inspired a strikingly gendered response as the themes of love and ghostly women became associated with the expedition. Male absence and female (spectral) presence became bound together in imaginative retellings of the Franklin disaster.' In Victorian Britain, as already shown in previous chapters, stories of women flitting between the material and supernatural realm proliferated both in fiction and in news reports of clairvoyants, ghostly experiments and seances. Women's supposed sensitivity made them more susceptible to psychic dreams and visions. Not only that, though: sensational tales of women reaching out to their loved ones stranded on the ice made for great melodrama. As McCorristine goes on to say, 'women were psychically connected to their male lovers across the cartographic divide, transgressing even the boundaries of what was natural in the physical world. Such was the power of this polar love to unite souls across space and time ...' For the average British person, far removed from the actual tragedy of the missing explorers, such heart-wrenching, nature-defying discussion was hard to resist.

Wilkie Collins, who, as we've already seen, had an interest in supernatural sleep, was clearly fascinated by the reports of the British public seeing the *Terror* and *Erebus* in their dreams. Collaborating with Charles Dickens, he wrote a play in 1856 called *The Frozen Deep*. Its life on the stage was short-lived, but Collins published the original novella – really just his quick summary of the plot – in 1885. Some of it is rather unabashed in its similarity to the Franklin expedition: its lost captain, for example, is literally called Frank. For the sake of drama, though, Collins adds a jealous crew member in Richard Wardour, who resents Frank for marrying the woman he also loves. Clara, Frank's wife, embodies both the desperate Lady Franklin and the phenomenon of women professing to be psychically linked to the lost crew. At one point, Clara falls into a clairvoyant sleep and has the following dream:

> A moment of silence follows, and in that moment the vision has changed. She sees [Frank] on the iceberg now, at the mercy of the bitterest enemy he has on earth. She sees him drifting: over the black water: through the ashy light.

'Wake, Frank! wake and defend yourself! Richard Wardour knows that I love you. Richard Wardour's vengeance will take your life! Wake, Frank – wake! You are drifting to your death!' A low groan of horror bursts from her, sinister and terrible to hear. 'Drifting! drifting!' she whispers to herself; 'drifting to his death!'[6]

The Frozen Deep aptly summarises the public's fascination with dreams of the Franklin expedition. It's a very distinct phenomenon, too – and certainly the most documented. It shows how our dream stories have been sources of (albeit false) hope for other people, and believed to be ways of communicating – even travelling – across the globe through sleep. While these attitudes don't have quite the same hold on our imagination today, one aspect of the Franklin dreams remains: dreams prey on our anxieties, making us live through situations that we dread.

☆ ☆ ☆

The relationship between dreams and stories was something that fascinated nineteenth-century thinkers. Dreams were sources of inspiration, the very foundations of fiction. But fiction could in turn provoke strange dreams, and thus the cycle continued. Robert Macnish, in *The Philosophy of Sleep* (1830), warned against the dangers of reading spooky stories before bed. 'If, for instance,' he says, 'we have been engaged in the perusal of such works as "The Monk," "The Mysteries of Udolpho," or "Satan's Invisible World Discovered;" and if an attack of nightmare should supervene, it will be aggravated into sevenfold horror by the spectral phantoms with which our minds have been thereby filled.

We will enter into all the fearful mysteries of these writings, which, instead of being mitigated by slumber, acquire an intensity which they never could have possessed in the waking state.'

Macnish goes further, though, and suggests that writers, students and philosophers are particularly susceptible to haunted sleep. He relates the sad story of the writer and physician John Polidori, contemporary of Coleridge and Byron and author of 'The Vampyre', who supposedly overdosed on laudanum in order to cure his persistent sleep paralysis (although the actual cause of his death has been contested). These kinds of people have bad digestion, Macnish says, because they have sedentary lifestyles and 'habits of intellectual or melancholy reflection' that provoke vivid and scary dreams. His cure of choice for such disturbed nights is to take 'the common blue pill'. Ironically, the main ingredient of this pill was mercury, which is highly poisonous and, in large enough quantities, can lead to insomnia, delirium and psychotic episodes.

This anxiety between fiction and dreams had a revival during the moral panic over comic books in 1950s America. Comic books and their content, particularly anything to do with horror and violence, no matter how tame we might consider them today, were condemned by members of the United States government for encouraging juvenile delinquency. Just as Macnish warned of Gothic stories frightening a reader, the social discussion around comics suggested that the dreams inspired by comic books could damage a child's mind. It was, however, hotly debated. In a record of a 1955 meeting of a subcommittee investigating juvenile delinquency in Nashville, Tennessee, we see the topic turn to the insidious evil of the comic. The members report giving a 'specimen' comic book to a middle-aged doctor, who 'told us he had nightmares after reading them'. Imagine, they say, what it will 'do to a child's mind'.[7] Five years earlier, however, an article in American magazine *Newsweek* actually defended comic-induced nightmares. According to so-called 'psychiatric experts', if a child has bad dreams caused by what they see in comic books, 'it is a good thing because it will draw attention to his real anxieties and difficulties'.[8] What we don't see, both in Macnish and the comic-book moral panic of the 1950s, is evidence that this was anything more than speculation. There are no specific examples of children having nightmares after reading *Superman*, or of members of the Victorian public suffering with troubled sleep after reading a gruesome story. It's more likely, perhaps, that these pandemics of bad dreams were used as a way to communicate the critic's personal preference for the content of literature.

A writer who welcomed dark and frightening dreams was Robert Louis Stevenson (1850–94), author of works such as 'The Strange Case of Dr Jekyll and Mr Hyde' and 'The Body Snatcher'. Several of Stevenson's stories are exactly the sort of thing Macnish warns against reading before bed; his stories are rife with Gothic imagery, decay, phantoms, vampires, the darkness lurking within us all.

In a collection of his essays, *Across the Plains* (1892), Stevenson includes 'A Chapter on Dreams'. He describes dreams as wonderful gifts, rather than twisted spectres brought on by overactive imaginations. He makes particular reference to his own dreams, which he often relies on to provide him with material to use in his writing. Stevenson has an odd but rather cute way of thinking about his dreams: he says they are created and populated by 'Little People', who 'do one-half my work for me while I am fast asleep, and in all human likelihood, do the rest for me as well, when I am wide awake and fondly suppose I do it for myself.'[9]

The Little People were responsible for many of the scenes in 'The Strange Case of Dr Jekyll and Mr Hyde'. This story is the infamous tale of a physician whose invention of a curious powder changes him from a timid man of science to a crude, hulking, violent criminal. But are the two personalities as separate as they first appear? Re-reading this story in light of Stevenson's interest in dreams gives it a new meaning. The lawyer investigating the case of a child seriously injured by Mr Hyde finds his sleep disturbed by his own imaginings of the crime. As Stevenson describes it: 'The figure ... haunted the lawyer all night; and if at any time he dozed over, it was but to see it glide more stealthily through sleeping houses, or move the more swiftly and still the more swiftly, even to dizziness, through wider labyrinths of lamplighted city, and at every street corner crush a child and leave her screaming.'[10]

The essence of the story – the duality of our personalities – is intriguing from the perspective of sleep. Stevenson presents Dr Jekyll as a nervous intellectual, and Hyde as an arrogant brute. But Hyde *is* Dr Jekyll, and we have to remember that Jekyll was the one who created, and took, the powder in the first place. Our dreams present something similar, if not quite as exaggerated as in Stevenson's story. In our dreams we are less inhibited, and our actions are often driven by impulse and instinct rather than rational judgement. If our dreams are especially vivid, we can see this duality clearly, even if it makes us uncomfortable. For example, I am much louder and brashly confident in my dreams, taking action quickly or swaggering my way through encounters with people I'd normally be shy in front of. We don't necessarily have an inner Hyde, but perhaps Stevenson is right in suggesting that there is a different side to us that lives in our dreams and nightmares.

☆ ☆ ☆

While the believed function and significance of dreams has changed, we remain fascinated and puzzled by these nightly dramas. In addition to the ever-increasing insight we're gaining into the operations of the brain, dreams continue to have cultural importance, particularly in terms of the *ways* we tell dreams. They are stories – little narratives that we shape and edit and embellish, ready to tell a friend in the pub or send over social media.

One of the most influential moments in the modern history of dream narratives was Sigmund Freud's *The Interpretation of Dreams*. First published in 1900, this book has become something of a cult classic, with Freud's likenesses appearing in films, cartoons and books to ponder over a character's nightmare for clues.

Freud is considered to be at the forefront of the psychoanalysis movement – a particularly popular way of understanding someone's mind through the interpretation of unconscious symbols and disguises. This is the foundation for *The Interpretation of Dreams*: a person's true thoughts, feelings and repressed memories can be unpicked through the abstract symbols and motifs in their dreams.

The main thesis of Freud's book is that dreams communicate our deepest, darkest desires. They are a form of 'wish fulfilment', as he calls it. This can be a very simple wish – Freud dreams about water because he is thirsty and desires a drink. Or, it can be a more emotional or sexual wish. Not being able to act on or discuss this wish produces mental distress in waking life. Dreams, according to Freud, are packed with clues to these wishes, but it is the role of the psychoanalyst to unmask the symbols and show them for what they really are.

One of the first dreams Freud uses to introduce his theory is one of his own. He experienced the dream in 1895, when he was treating a young widow named Irma, a family friend, through psychoanalysis. His dream is extremely creepy and seems to fixate on the body:

> A great hall – a number of guests, whom we are receiving – among them Irma, whom I immediately take aside, as though to answer her letter, and to reproach her for not yet accepting the 'solution'. I say to her: 'If you still have pains, it is really only your own fault.' – She answers: 'If you knew what pains I have now in the throat, stomach, and abdomen – I am choked by them.' I am startled, and look at her. She looks pale and puffy. I think that after all I must be overlooking some organic affection. I take her to the window and look into her throat. She offers some resistance to this, like a woman who has a set of false teeth. I think, surely, she doesn't need them. – The mouth then opens wide, and I find a large white spot on the right, and elsewhere I see extensive greyish-white scabs adhering to curiously curled formations, which are evidently shaped like the turbinal bones of the nose. – I quickly call Dr M., who repeats the examination and confirms it … Dr M. looks quite unlike his usual self; he is very pale, he limps, and his chin is clean-shaven … Now my friend Otto, too, is standing beside her, and my friend

Leopold percusses her covered chest, and says: 'She has a dullness below, on the left,' and also calls attention to an infiltrated portion of skin on the left shoulder (which I can feel, in spite of the dress) ... M. says: 'There's no doubt that it's an infection, but it doesn't matter; dysentery will follow and the poison will be eliminated.' ... We know, too, precisely how the infection originated. My friend Otto, not long ago, gave her, when she was feeling unwell, an injection of a preparation of [...] propionic acid ... trimethylamine (the formula of which I see before me, printed in heavy type) ... One doesn't give such injections so rashly ... Probably, too, the syringe was not clean.[11]

Freud then dissects certain phrases of his dream, compartmentalising them into symbols and ideas. The dream is subject to a literary analysis, just as I might get students to do in a seminar. He pauses particularly on the inclusion of dysentery in his dream, wondering if he was recalling other illnesses from patients and his family. 'Dysentery suggests something else,' Freud thinks, and concludes that it is similar to a previous case where the malady of the era, hysteria, seemed to mimic some of the symptoms of dysentery. He ends his analysis by uncovering his wish: that he could blame someone else – in the dream, it manifests through Otto – for the fact that Irma still wasn't cured of what ailed her.

Even though Freud's theories of wish fulfilment and psychoanalysis have been contested since the publication of *The Interpretation of Dreams*, it marks an important moment in modern dream-telling. He encouraged people to pay attention not simply to the images and sounds and sensations of dreams, but also to *how* they tell a dream to another person. He focused on the language used, and the self-censorship. What does it say about us that, when we describe a dream, we choose to miss out some of the more intimate or morally questionable elements and focus only on the amusing and strange? Dreams are intensely personal, but when we tell them to people, when we turn them into stories, we repackage them so that they fit a narrative model that is sure to be a crowd-pleaser.

The impact of Freud's work was far-reaching, not least in psychoanalytic circles. In the Golden Era of Hollywood in the 1940s and 50s, numerous plots featured aspects of his dream theories. Movies have often been compared to dreams. They can be abstract, full of symbols and references and cameos, complex situations and stories simplified into a smaller space, plunging you into a situation and not letting go until it's over. Like a nightmare, you find yourself chewing over the experience for hours or even days afterwards. Flashes of what you saw come back to haunt you, or make you laugh. And sometimes they really, *really* don't make sense.

One of the most notable uses of Freud's dream theories as a plot device is in Alfred Hitchcock's 1945 thriller, *Spellbound*. Ingrid Bergman stars as psychoanalyst Dr Constance Petersen, working in a hospital with rather questionable professional standards.[12] The hospital's old director is replaced with the dashing Gregory Peck as Dr Anthony Edwardes, but it soon becomes clear that Edwardes isn't who he says he is, can't remember who he is, and that the *real* Edwardes has been murdered. When this is revealed, Petersen and 'Edwardes' have already fallen in love via a brisk countryside walk and liverwurst sandwiches (the most romantic of all processed sandwich meats!), and Petersen is determined to prove that the impostor isn't the murderer of the real Dr Edwardes.

Later in the film, Petersen takes 'Edwardes', now using the pseudonym John Brown, to see her old mentor, a Freud-like psychoanalyst with a particular interest in dreams. He asks the possible impostor to recall a recent dream, and the audience is taken directly into Brown's sleeping mind.

The Spanish surrealist painter Salvador Dalí was brought in to design and direct this dream. Dalí himself had a keen interest in the liminal states of sleep and wakefulness, and several of his paintings are inspired and influenced by the bizarre imagery of the unconscious mind. His 1944 painting, 'Dream Caused by the Flight of a Bee Around a Pomegranate a Second Before Awakening',[13] for example, features a naked, reclining woman being set upon by a bayonet and tigers emerging from the mouth of a fish, which in turn springs from an open pomegranate. While this is a piece of static art, rather than a written narrative, it still aims to pin down the story of a dream. There's movement in the animals springing towards the woman, and in the background a spider-legged elephant teeters precariously, threatening to topple into the water below at any moment.

According to Ingrid Bergman, Dalí's original dream sequence in *Spellbound* was over twenty minutes long. If you've seen the film, you'll know that the two minutes that *did* make the cut are more than baffling and intense. All forms of dream-representation in fiction and art are fascinating, but the *Spellbound* dream packs quite a punch.

It opens in a peculiar casino, with giant, melting eyes decorating the curtains around the room. There is an attractive woman in a revealing dress kissing the other clients, showing

Brown's desire for the otherwise prim and proper Petersen. A man walks around with a giant pair of scissors, slicing through the eyes on the curtains. Brown is playing cards on a nauseatingly distorted card table, and the man he's playing against is suddenly accused of cheating by the owner, who is wearing a cloth mask that entirely covers and obscures his head. The scene then changes; Brown's card partner leaps from a high building while the casino owner stands behind, holding a wobbly wheel in Salvador Dalí's signature surrealist style. Brown then finds himself running down a huge, flat slope like the side of a pyramid, while a pair of dark wings chases after him.

The dream is interpreted using Freudian terms, of abstract and compressed memories and desires; they should be analysed in terms of symbols, and the symbols should be analysed in terms of what they disguise or distort. The climax of the film involves Petersen solving the puzzle of Brown's dream. He didn't murder Edwardes, but he witnessed it, and his dream is the compressed, twisted version of his memory. The casino, she realises, is the hospital, and Brown's card partner is Edwardes. They were having lunch together at a ski resort, when they were confronted by the 'casino proprietor' – the old director of the hospital, Dr Murchison. Angered at being forcefully replaced due to his age, Murchison, while Edwardes and Brown are on the ski slope, shoots Edwardes in the back. Edwardes falls off the precipice, just as the card partner in Brown's dream jumps from the building while the proprietor looks on behind. The wheel held by the proprietor in the dream, Petersen concludes, is the compressed symbol for 'revolver', the murder weapon.

The reason Brown is so profoundly upset by this, besides being the witness to a murder, is a result of unresolved childhood trauma. Throughout the film, Brown is shown to have a visceral reaction whenever he sees parallel lines: when Petersen traces her fork down a tablecloth, and by the stripes on her dressing gown. During his session of psychoanalysis, it is revealed that when he and his brother were children, he caused his brother's death by accidentally pushing him off a sloped wall and onto a spiked railing. The act of sliding down a slope and witnessing a gruesome death is mirrored in the murder at the ski resort, and the fresh trauma mingles with historic trauma to produce Brown's deep repression of memory.

☆　☆　☆

For me, dreams have been an important part of my life since childhood. They have always been multi-sensory, tactile and physical as well as colourful and detailed. If something happens to my body in a dream, like getting attacked by an animal, for example, I still feel a tingling sensation in that spot when I wake up. Some dreams profoundly affected me when I was growing up, and now my dreams are often the gateway into some of my strange sleep experiences.

A couple of years after my recurring dreams about a tin man (discussed in Chapter 1), I had a nightmare that was so awful it took me many months to get over. I'll say this now to get the laughter out of the way: this dream gave me a phobia of aliens. 'How can you have a phobia of aliens?' is usually the giggled question I have to answer when I reveal this ridiculous fact about myself. It's probably not unlike coulrophobia – the fear of clowns. My phobia is very specific to the 'little grey men' style of alien: spindly legs and a large, lemon-shaped head.

This dream happened around the year 2000, when I remember these bastards being everywhere. The millennium seemed dominated by a space-age aesthetic of UFOs and aliens.

The dream began in my primary school – a frequent site of my dreams, even now. It was a small school in my village; it's had a fancy extension now, but at the time it was a simple Victorian building with a long corridor going right the way through it. I was fascinated by this corridor, with its wooden floor resembling interlocking teeth and glazed brown wall tiles. It seemed about a mile long when I was a child, which makes it quite fertile ground for those stressful dreams where the room around you stretches on for ever. In the dream, I was standing in this corridor, looking at an old 1960s television set that had appeared in the foyer. It was night, but there was some sort of event happening at the school and I couldn't hear the television over the noise of people around me. I could see the screen clearly, though, and I was the only one taking notice of it.

A black-and-white picture showed an open plain with mountains in the distance. Above, in the sky, was a fuzzy grey disc wobbling unsteadily. The camera zoomed in; the UFO dominated the screen, and green and red lights erupted from the monochrome image.

The scene changed. I was at home, tucked up in my bed. There was a noise; the window to the left of me opened, and my Winnie the Pooh curtains billowed in the draught. A man dressed in a tweed suit floated into my room, legs slightly tucked under him as though he was kneeling on an invisible cushion. I wasn't scared at first, because he looked like Mr Majeika, the titular character from Humphrey Carpenter's series of children's books – one of my favourites. But I don't think I read them again after this dream.

The man continued his slow, underwater journey until he was hovering above my bed. He came to a stop and looked down at me. Just as I was beginning to feel a sense of danger, the man underwent a hideous transformation. I don't remember too much about this, because it happened so quickly, but there was a terrible ripping sound of cloth, skin, flesh, as though the alien was bursting out of the man's body. Something lunged towards me, and I saw teeth.

I woke up in a state. This was worse than any tin-man dream, or any nightmare I had had before. I remember running downstairs, clinging to the last rod of the baluster for strength, crying like I'd never cried before.

I wouldn't go back to bed. I couldn't. My parents and sisters tried to tell me that it was a dream, that it wasn't real, but that didn't make a difference. Perhaps I was well aware that it wasn't real, but it had scared me so badly and it felt real while it was happening. I think *because* it was vivid beyond any dream I'd previously experienced, to the point where I can still recall it clearly twenty-odd years later, I couldn't quite make the separation between fantasy and reality.

I wonder now, actually, if this alien-dream was a very early and one-off episode of sleep paralysis. It certainly shares some characteristics, not least because it seemed to happen rather early into the night, while my parents were still in the living room watching television.

My bedroom at night became a site of paralysing terror. I had to decamp into the bottom level of my sister's bunk bed. She wasn't pleased. And I wouldn't go back into my own room for several months. I couldn't even go *upstairs* alone when the rooms were dark. Every time I tried to go to sleep, all I could think about was that aliens were creeping into my room. They had morphed from the floating, fanged monstrosity I saw in my dream into the little grey men of pop-culture iconography. Even now, I cringe when I see anything to do with UFOs.

We tried a lot of things to get me over the fear of the dark. Finally, my parents decided that perhaps rearranging my little room would help. They bought me a new bed, raised high off the floor so you could fit a desk in underneath. Perhaps the aliens wouldn't be able to negotiate the ladder, I thought. I had a nightlight on a shelf next to my new bed, though, and when I thought everyone had gone to bed I would turn it on and leave it glowing all night.

By this time, I had relinquished Doggy to teddy bear heaven (a shoebox in my wardrobe – I refused to get rid of him completely) and replaced him with the valiant Alfred, a large giraffe I bought on my birthday in Chester Zoo. He was about the size of my torso – probably still an accurate measurement because I don't think I've grown since I bought him – and in an upright sitting position which meant I could wrap his legs around my stomach in a hug. I would sleep facing the wall, back turned to the door, clutching Alfred like this so his head peeked over my shoulder. I told him to tell me if any aliens appeared; he promised he would. He would stay vigilant, all night, and I would trust him to warn me, defend me, if those little grey men I feared so much came into the room.

I still have Alfred; I feel like we've been through many rough times together. The way I sleep, on my side and with my hands tucked up across my shoulders, is still the shape from this time of my life, except Alfred is back at my parents' house rather than squished up against my chest. I always take a moment to say hello to him whenever I visit, though.

Eventually, I got over my fear. It was a very slow process, not helped by the time I decided to watch M. Night Shyamalan's 2002 film about aliens, *Signs*, as some sort of exposure therapy. If I could make it through the film, thought nine-year-old me, I would be officially cured of my fear. I did not make it through the film.

☆ ☆ ☆

In the mid-twentieth century, when the public imagination was still buzzing with Freud's ideas of dream interpretation and psychoanalysis, there was a flurry of activity to pin down the experience of dreams in both scientific understanding and in art and writing. Sleep clinics were developed to investigate disorders such as insomnia and narcolepsy, and swathes of surveys were done to investigate dreams. One of these surveys investigated the aspect of colour, and whether people were more likely to dream in monochrome. In recent years, the results have been looked at again, and the survey repeated, to form a very different picture that suggests dreaming and art are more linked than previously thought. More specifically, it showed a relationship between the colours of dreams and the kinds of film and television we watch.

When I was a child, I remember hearing people say that we only dreamed in black-and-white. I thought, therefore, that I must be very special because my dreams were always in bright, clear colour. The idea that we don't dream in colour is a myth, and one that was perpetuated by the generations of people who grew up in the early- to mid-twentieth century. In other words, those who grew up watching black-and-white movies and television. Between the 1940s and late 1950s, when monochromatic media proliferated and glorious Technicolour was still rare, numerous surveys were conducted into the presence of colour in dreams, and they found low results – 29%, 15%, even as low as 9% of sample groups reported dreams in colour. However, once the silver screen exploded with psychedelic rainbows in the 1960s, the survey results suddenly showed that the vast *majority*, not the minority, of participants said they perceived colour in their dreams.[14]

Connected with this, a weird thing has been happening to me recently. I've become a bit obsessed with 1940s Hollywood, and I'll watch one or two films a week from this period. I especially like Bette Davis, with her moon-bright eyes, so it was inevitable that I would dream about her at some point. When she did appear, it was peculiar: she was an ash-coloured figure in an otherwise vibrant outdoor scene. I could see green grass and the pale blue of the sky, but there was Bette Davis in every shade of grey. It was a fragment of a dream, but I pondered over it for a long time. I could understand how consuming nothing *but* black-and-white media might slowly sap the colours from a dream, maybe even permanently.

Another phenomenon that perhaps arose from the impact of *The Interpretation of Dreams* was the sudden popularity of the published dream diaries of notable writers and cultural figures. Federico Fellini, the famous Italian director of such films as *La Dolce Vita* (1960), kept an extensive dream diary with notes accompanying strange, lurid drawings. Jack Kerouac, author of *On the Road*, published his collection of dreams and thoughts, which he recorded immediately after waking. Titled *Book of Dreams* (1961), it's a strange, messy, often frantic spill of

thoughts and images. Some dreams finish mid-sentence, sometimes mid-word, written out exactly as Kerouac scribbled them
down. Here's a typical example:

> Wild as seen from the top of a grassy hill outside town,
> it's Mexico city, where are elephant water holes, funny
> shepherds, me with a huge well not huge medium sized
> bag of tea in which I'm running my hand as though
> through gold but it's just weed, and the day's bright,
> flowing clouds, the Plateau North of the Great America
> of the World is fine and white like a beard of a patriarch
> in the Popocatepetl Sky – my silk and lace – able you
> – Events –[15]

Kerouac's presentation of his dreams is comparable to some of
Salvador Dalí's dream-like paintings, which have their roots in
the experiences of dreams but are far more exaggerated and styl-
ised than what we normally encounter.

William S. Burroughs, Kerouac's contemporary and friend,
published *My Education: A Book of Dreams* in 1995, two years
before his death. It's fascinating to see how differently the two
writers narrate their dreams. There is a simplicity to Burroughs'
dreams; they read in the same way as you would tell a dream
to someone standing next to you – there is a little confusion,
some self-analysis, but they are otherwise packaged in a neat
and readable narrative. And they are, for the most part, incredibly mundane. Dreams aren't always explosive, violent, dazzling
rides through some mystical realm – sometimes they can simply be about wandering around a beige hotel in search of your
wallet – but that doesn't mean they can't be turned into stories

or art. This is how Burroughs presents his dreams: there's no particular sense of embellishment, but they're still intriguing to read in their own right.

Because of the ordinariness but also the clarity with which Burroughs presents his dreams, we get a good sense of his waking experiences. We could probably guess at what he got up to over the last few days from the scenarios presented in some of his more detailed dreams. There are repeated mentions of people from his life, and, perhaps more importantly, personal, recurring symbols. Burroughs often dreamt about cats. A lot. Here's a good example:

> I am looking for a place to shave. I live in a cubicle room with three cats and there is a rusty basin with a cold-water tap. I decide to shave at Allen Ginsberg's, which is just up the street. A maze of streets, rooms, corridors, cul-de-sacs, doorways so narrow one must squeeze through sideways, huge open courtyards and rooms. I decide to take two cats to Allen's place, which consists of a bath-tub in a small room. I can shave using the bathtub. Look around to find my cats are gone. I reach under the bathtub and pull out a long, thin gray cat but can't find my cats. Is there an opening? I should have left them at home.[16]

The cats in his dreams always seem to represent some sort of anxiety. When he dreams about his own cats, they go missing, become ill, or suddenly act out of character and scratch Burroughs. Sometimes, though, he dreams about cats he doesn't recognise, and they seem to be objects of fear.

A haunted room. I am attacked by a cat that turns into
a ghost and bites. Then I see a small orange cat by my
head on the pillow. I tell someone I will not sleep there
again. Go up in an elevator to another apartment.

Animals in general feature in a great deal of Burroughs' dreams
in *My Education*. There are theories that they represent fear –
it is a re-emergence of our primitive anxieties of being mauled
and bitten by predators and poisonous vermin. The cats in
Burroughs' dreams are fascinating, though. There always seems
to be an associated fear with them: fear of betrayal, abandonment
or encountering unfamiliar cats that are hostile towards him.

My parents have a cat, a little tuxedo-patterned chap called
Mow who turned up in the garden one day as a malnourished
stray and never left. I don't dream about him often, but when I do
he always has a strange trait: he talks. This is probably my own
fault for narrating his thoughts whenever I'm visiting (at least I
make myself laugh), but it's odd that my dreams turn him into a
character who gives me advice or a warning or discusses whatever
situation is going on. Sometimes, too, I dream about tiny, sad,
abandoned kittens that I find in random places: in my pocket,
in the washing machine, dropped on my head by a passing bird.
I blame these on the proliferation of vapid animal-rescue videos
that the Facebook algorithm endlessly pushes into my face. I don't
think these dreams happen often enough to be recurring, though,
at least not in the way that they do for Burroughs. I dream a lot
about trains and stations; the subject and theme of the dreams
are always different, but I would say that was my biggest recurring motif. It's interesting that we all have our own set of symbols
and motifs that make up the fabric of our dreams.

It's not unusual, of course, for people to keep dream diaries, but the twentieth-century cultural phenomenon of the published dream diary – in its entirety, and not as a section in a collected book of letters or notes – suggests the popularity and interest in seeing writers and artists lend their distinctive style to the effort of presenting dreams in waking life. Just as our dreams are unique in their appearance and tropes, so too is the way in which we attempt to describe them.

☆ ☆ ☆

Meredith has never been anything other than an antagonist in my dreams. What has changed the most is me. In my teenage years and into my early twenties, when we were still in contact with each other, she was the aggressor, the villain, always one step ahead of me. I was anxious, weak, unable to break out of the mixture of jealousy and loyalty she was trying to make me feel. I'd wake up ashamed of myself.

My dreams of her these days have become more exaggerated. As I've described a few times in this book, it's no longer a true picture of Meredith that I see, but something that has been exacerbated because of the way she has haunted my sleep since I was an adolescent. I now have two distinct types of dream about Meredith.

The first kind is dominated by fear. These usually turn into sleep paralysis or a lucid dream. Here's an example: the mobile phone I had in high school was a little green Nokia, and in the dream I was showing it to a man and a woman wearing white lab coats. They were reading a string of texts from Meredith (I made sure to highlight the one where she called me a 'nymph'). In the next moment, she had appeared, and was ferociously trying to snatch the phone from me. She pushed me onto my back, and I woke to a strange, half-dreaming sleep paralysis episode in which I thought she was dragging me down my mattress by the ankles.

The other type of dream doesn't particularly make me feel any better in the morning, but I suppose it's an improvement of sorts. These dreams are angry. Very angry. Nordic heavy metal angry. I hate confrontation of all kinds; in the same way as when I'm afraid, I just go very quiet when something is upsetting me. Not so in my dreams.

On one occasion, I dreamt that I was waiting for my train at Euston station. It was crowded; people were swarming around me and, because of my height, I couldn't see over their shoulders.

I ducked and dodged my way through until I reached a quieter spot where I could see the display boards. Where was the train to Chester? I scanned across the constantly changing amber letters and symbols. Found it. Platform 47. Where was that? People surged past me, filing through like sand in an egg timer towards the corridor in front. I became part of the crowd, letting them sweep me along towards the platform.

I was getting closer and closer to a group of people standing by the wall. One of them broke away, and stood staring at me.

Meredith.

No no no no. The crowd was carrying me forwards and I couldn't grip the floor with my feet. I couldn't stop myself. She waited patiently for me to be delivered to her.

Her fingernails, sharp and painted gold, dug into my wrist as she pulled me out of the stream of people. She led me over to a bench, and we sat down. For a moment, I felt very young. But only for a moment.

'We need to talk,' she said.

My chest burned; I tore my wrist away. 'I have *nothing* to say to you,' I yelled, every word as crisp and fanged as a hissing cat. I tried to get up, but her hand was like a concrete block and she wrenched me back down.

'Please, Alice.'

'Talk about what? My train's about to leave. I can't *do* this now, Meredith.'

'We need to talk.' Her eyes were glittering. 'You shut me out. How could you do that? Don't you know how much you've hurt me?'

The guilt stung, and I stopped resisting her hand. But only for a moment. I was angry before, but now it felt as though my ribcage was splitting open. I started to shout, to *scream* at her, louder and louder. 'You know what you did! You crossed boundaries! Are you *listening* to me? You *know* what you did. You made me think I was going mad! You told me to get therapy. You know what you did.'

Her grip tightened on my wrist and I wondered if she would snap my bones.

But she didn't say anything. She stared at me as though she didn't understand the language I was speaking. Her expression was cold. She didn't care.

My shoulders sagged; my rage was spent. I quietly told her I needed to catch my train. She let me go.

I dream of movement and escape more than anything else. I'm always trying to leave, to get somewhere, and things are getting in my way. I have to get out by any means possible, so I have quite a lot of dreams where I'm squeezing my body through the few inches' gap in an open window or, more strangely, attempting to force my way through a wall as though it's made of surgical rubber. The tin-man dreams were a precursor to these, but that was always in wide open spaces. These days, I dream about having to get out of rooms. Tiny, menacing, cold spaces with locked doors and small windows.

Meredith made closed spaces seem threatening, from the corridor leading up to the blue door of her classroom to the claustrophobic darkness of the drama studio. I used to feel sick to my stomach in her presence, but I told myself it was just shyness; again, my body always knew what was up.

In the few years after I knew her, particularly during my undergraduate degree, I suffered with a particular anxiety that, handily, made me terrified of lecture theatres and seminar rooms. I soldiered through it, but I think there were a few occasions where I probably annoyed my friends by insisting on sitting at the end of a row or at a table near the exit. Even so, sometimes I would still spend the lecture trying my best to listen while subduing a storm of nausea and panic. I had to be closest to the door – a sad parallel to Meredith's cunning seating plan where I was always the last to leave, escape blocked by her arm stretched across the open doorway.

I calmed down a lot during my PhD, and now I teach in lecture theatres and crammed seminar rooms without feeling any of those old churnings in my stomach. Nevertheless, fleeing is still a recurring theme. Unlike my childhood nightmares, though, it's not my life that's in danger, but my freedom. I know I'm not going to be killed; it's the feeling of hands closing around me, of being singled out and coveted.

Meredith singled me out from the start, and did it under the guise of being helpful. In the first few weeks of the school year, she kept me behind to give me feedback on an essay. 'I'll do this with everyone,' she said, which turned out to be a big old lie when I asked a few of my friends in the class about it.

A few months later, the school librarian suddenly handed in her notice and left. There was a period of a week or two before the replacement could start. One afternoon, another English teacher found me at lunchtime. She explained the situation, and said that Meredith would be stepping in.

'But she'll only do it if you help her,' she said.

I remember this phrase clearly. It wasn't that Meredith suggested I help her, or thought I'd enjoy helping, or even that it was high time I actually did something as Head Girl besides wear a nice badge. No, she'd *only* do it if I helped her, and it all hinged on my compliance. Now, I love libraries and librarians in all their glorious forms, but I really do think we as a school could have survived being cast adrift from the four old computers and half a dozen shelves of *Animorphs* books for a week. Who knows, perhaps this was just the other teacher's wording and not what Meredith actually said, but this was the kind of thing she had done before. Nothing particularly bad happened in the library; I remember sitting behind the desk with her at lunch in the otherwise empty room. She offered me some of her crisps, and said I was as quiet as a mouse, and then the week was over and the new librarian started work.

I tried to be rebellious sometimes, which in any situation is near-impossible for me. I would dash out of the classroom like a weasel with an overstuffed backpack; I would try my best to stay away from Meredith. But there were always books of hers in my bedroom that I needed to give back, and she'd got into my head so much that I found I couldn't *not* see her, even though a growing part of me desperately wanted to run far away. I think she picked up on this, though, because she seemed to make an effort to make me jealous by telling me about how marvellous and wonderful other, younger, more malleable students were. She would point them out or show me their work or tell me which books she had let *them* borrow. And, being an angsty teenager in need of attention, I would then try to be better. It completely churned me up inside, because no matter how many times I told myself to avoid her, I somehow still ended up in her classroom after school. It wasn't purely out of manipulation, either: I was scared of her doing to other students what she was doing to me. Particularly after I left that school and went to college, I thought that if I did what she wanted, she wouldn't move on to some other naive girl. It took me a long time to let go of this anxiety and realise that I wasn't responsible for them or for her.

My dreams often feature this theme of being made to do something in order to save other people. I've been singled out, separated from a group, and their safety depends on my obedience to some sort of authority figure. Sometimes it's in a strange context, far removed from high school, but quite often Meredith is at the heart of it all. Looking through my dream diary, a lot of entries involve her urging me to do something I don't want to do, and how others will suffer if I don't bow to her whims.

On 9 March 2018 I had the following dream.

I was in a large, dilapidated mansion – like Miss Havisham's house in Charles Dickens' *Great Expectations*. Sunshine was streaming through the windows, but the interior was dark, cluttered and dusty. I was there with a group of my friends, but we were otherwise alone in the house. We had decided to play hide-and-seek, as I'm sure any group of adults *would* do in this sort of situation, and I was going first as the seeker.

We were in a room with big bay windows and lots of alcoves and hiding spaces. Tattered sheets were draped over bits of furniture, and there were bits of broken wood, old paintings, and other junk strewn across the floor. I carefully picked my way over to an alcove while my friends scampered out of the door.

I began to count to one hundred. 'One ... two ... three ...'

There was a creaking noise near the door. A piece of furniture shifted.

'Ten ... eleven ...'

Someone was creeping up behind me. My stomach sank; it wasn't one of my friends, I could sense it. They came closer and closer, and then I knew. It was Meredith. I tried to ignore her. I continued to count with an almost aggressive determination.

'*Eighteen ... nineteen ... twenty ...*'

'Alice.'

The sound of her voice saying my name was like a handful of snow melting down my back. I moved away from the wall and lifted my hands from my eyes.

'What?' I asked, trying to sound as annoyed and confident as I could, but the word still wobbled in my throat.

She looked calm; the master of the situation, as always. She had her hand behind her back, and she slowly brought it round to show me what she was hiding.

It was a glass bottle, unlabelled, half-full of a suspicious, dark liquid. It looked like rum, but I was sure it wasn't.

She held it out to me, with a shot-glass in her other hand.

'What is that?' I said, shifting now to get a little bit of distance between us.

She only moved closer to fill the gap. She shook the bottle. 'I want you to have some. It's fine; I'm giving it to everyone else when I find them, but you're the first person I've seen.'

I looked around the room; suddenly a couple of my friends had returned, milling around as though they had forgotten the game. I wondered why Meredith had just said what she'd said, when there were other people here with us now.

'Everyone else is going to get some.'

'I don't want any,' I said.

She moved closer, thrusting the bottle at me. 'Yes, you do.'

The others in the room weren't looking at me. They weren't going to help, even if I called out. I was suddenly very afraid of Meredith, and the drink she was holding. I knew there was nothing I could do; I wasn't strong or big enough to force my way past her, out of this alcove.

I nodded, and held out a shaking hand.

Meredith seemed pleased; she poured me a shot and handed it to me. I drank it down, and woke up.

☆ ☆ ☆

Dreams may have evolved to deliberately present us with threatening experiences. This is the basis of a theory proposed by neuroscientist Antti Revonsuo in a 2000 article titled 'The Reinterpretation of Dreams'. Revonsuo analyses past and present theories about the function and purpose of dreams. He disregards Freud's wish-fulfilment theory, and also argues against Freud's later idea, posed in revised editions of *Beyond the Pleasure Principle*, that dreams repeat unpleasant or repressed memories until they lose their initial emotional impact.[17] Regarding the latter, Revonsuo criticises the idea by pointing out how often this function 'deserts us when we need it most'.[18]

But can we accept that there is no purpose or reason for dreaming? Revonsuo says not. If this *were* the case, he points out that dreams would be far more messy and unrelated to our daily experiences. They would be more like a series of those jarring magic-eye pictures than a clear, if peculiar, unfolding narrative. He wonders about the evolution of the brain in accordance with the environment of early humans. Other researchers have shown that the dreaming brain does operate in a rather primitive way; dreams are the closest we come to operating like our mammalian cousins and ancestors, living in the moment and adapting to whatever the current situation demands, regardless of what has already happened or what will happen in a few moments' time.

In this respect, then, dreams take us back to a time when our brains were constantly alert and ready to react to danger. We might have dreams about being unprepared for a school exam decades after we left, or standing on a stage and realising we're not wearing clothes, but isn't that a rather primitive fear? Anxiety dreams are often about being unprepared and vulnerable to danger, not unlike being faced with a dangerous animal or catastrophic weather and not having the tools or foresight to protect ourselves. This is Revonsuo's theory: dreams are a lingering, archaic process left over from when we faced potentially life-threatening situations on a daily basis.

By dreaming about being without a weapon and cornered by a predator, the sleeper rehearses survival tactics but is also given a reminder of why it is so important to take precautions. The next day, they will take their weapon with them, or they will have a plan as to what to do if their dream became a reality. Children's dreams, according to Revonsuo, depict much more basic needs and direct threats to safety than the dreams of adults.

In tribes and communities across the globe where there is a more pronounced risk of dangers from the natural world – such as poisonous snakes, large predatory mammals, forest fires – there is still evidence of the usefulness of this theory of dreams. Revonsuo discusses the work of several anthropologists, showing how the dreams of tribal societies still seem to function in a way that prepares them for the real dangers they face in their everyday lives. A good example is the work of Thomas Gregor, who studied the Mehinaku tribe in central Brazil.[19]

Gregor took a survey of 385 dreams reported by the Mehinaku community. For them, dreams have a great significance, and often serve as predictions and warnings. The Mehinaku, as reported by Gregor, believe that the soul (or 'shadow') leaves the body in sleep via the iris of the eye and travels through a 'nocturnal world peopled by spirits, monsters, and the souls of other sleeping villagers'. It is a common morning practice to tell others about the dreams experienced in the night, not just for conversation but for assistance in decoding any symbols that represent danger.

What Gregor found was that there was a high prevalence of animal dreams among the Mehinaku. Animals represented the most common danger, either in their own right or as symbols of another disaster. To dream of a swarm of flying ants, for example, warned of a sudden death in the family. Animals and people in Mehinaku dreams are intertwined; there is a sense of transformation in many of the anecdotes, of people becoming animals – showing the hidden danger of an individual – or an animal can turn into a human, de-escalating the situation.

One of the most interesting aspects of Gregor's study was the gender disparity in the subjects and symbols of the community's dreams. While the theme of being attacked by an animal was common to both men and women, the *type* of animals differed significantly. For women, who in this tribe were largely unarmed and unused to confrontation with more powerful predators, nightmares involved vicious dogs, boar or wild cats native to the area such as jaguars. However, for the men there was a sense of being prepared to face such dangers. They confronted them regularly, and had years of experience in wielding weapons and hunting. Their dreams still featured the above animals, but not as regularly and with a reduced sense of anxiety and danger. Instead, the dreams that most disturbed the men of the Mehinaku tribe were the more subtle, undetectable threats such as spiders, snakes, and other poisonous creatures. You can face a snarling jaguar head-on if you have the bravery, strength, and a good weapon, but nothing can save you from an unseen snake lunging out of the undergrowth and fatally biting your ankle.

But Gregor also found an unexpected and insidious element to the dreams of the Mehinaku. He discovered an increasing prevalence of nightmares relating to being invaded and assaulted by urban-dwelling Brazilians. Specifically, both the men and women of the village dreamt of being sexually assaulted by Brazilian men. For the Mehinaku, this scenario was as vivid an anxiety to them as their dreams of being attacked by a powerful or poisonous animal.

Gregor makes a fascinating case here for the use of dream collection and analysis as a key anthropological tool. We can learn so much about the lives of communities through the themes and content of their dreams. But it also bolsters Revonsuo's theory that dreams prepare us for dangerous situations, and that they are a safe place for us to rehearse our reactions and tactics when confronted with conflict.

☆　☆　☆

In the first few weeks of 2020, news of a novel coronavirus strain found in China started to appear around the world. By early March, cases in the UK were creeping steadily upwards, and by the end of the month, we joined several countries in entering a major national lockdown. There were innumerable implications at this early and strange stage of the pandemic, from overwhelming work and domestic pressures, loss of loved ones, and long-term loss of health, to reconnecting with nature, finding new hobbies and baking lots of banana bread.

Perhaps one of the more unexpected consequences of the start of the pandemic was how it affected our sleep. For some people, the anxiety of the situation led to insomnia. For others, particularly those whose alarm normally woke them up early to begin their commute, working or learning from home meant they could sleep later, into stages of REM sleep that would usually be cut short. As a result, they were experiencing long, vivid dreams such as they hadn't known for a long time. News reports about this phenomenon were frequent: in *The Guardian*, for example, three articles on so-called 'lockdown dreaming' appeared online in the space of eleven days in April 2020.[20] Our collective experience of the pandemic – especially for people such as frontline health workers and other key workers facing the worst of the situation – was traumatic, and will likely continue to provide material for our nightmares for years to come.

Surveys and research into pandemic dreams began as soon as the phenomenon was noticed, and further work is still being done. An early study was published in 2020 by Cassidy MacKay and Teresa L. DeCicco at Trent University, Canada. MacKay told me she was working on her undergraduate thesis project under DeCicco's supervision, which involved conducting a dream journal experiment to see 'whether experiencing emotional abuse from a romantic partner had an effect on an individual's dream content.' The project began on 24 February 2020, but was cut short on 12 March when Trent University – like many organisations – closed its doors to students and switched to remote learning. While MacKay's original project had to be cancelled, she and DeCicco did find something interesting in the data they managed to collect. The pandemic was directly influencing the participants' sleep.

They found distinct changes in the recorded dreams in line with what they'd expect from people who reported generalised anxiety in their waking hours. In terms of content, the participants suddenly began to see recurrent images, some in common with each other. Animals cropped up more regularly than before, as well as food imagery, which might have reflected the panic-buying and hoarding of supplies seen in several countries.[21] Additionally, many participants' dreams now focused, unusually, on heads. The sudden global proliferation of images regarding the head – the coughing and spreading of germs, the face masks, the slack mouths of patients on ventilators – seems to have seeped into the dream lives of many of these participants. While the study involved a small group of only nineteen, the anecdotes and data generated paint an interesting picture of how the pandemic slowly started taking over people's dreams.

A similar, but larger, study was conducted by a team in Italy. Led by Serena Scarpelli, the researchers surveyed a sample of nearly 6,000 adult Italians. An interesting finding of this study was that the participants whose lifestyles had changed the most, in terms of their working or learning situation and the amount of time spent sleeping, also experienced the greatest increase in emotional intensity in their dreams compared to their pre-COVID dreams.[22] Scarpelli's team conclude their study by encouraging further investigation, not treating the pandemic dreams as an interesting novelty, but examining their clinical implications and possible treatment. In some articles on the subject, mostly those in popular journalism, there was a sense that these dreams were a bit of light curiosity, but I agree with Scarpelli that it needs to be taken more seriously than that. For a lot of people, it will be a way of trauma manifesting itself, and it might seriously impact their waking lives unless we respect and try to understand these dreams – and find a way to ease them.

This is part of the work of Deborah Bryon, a psychoanalyst from Denver, USA. She theorises that the common negative content in people's dreams at the height of the pandemic was partly due to a shift in our perspective of time. In short, our plans for the next few months of our lives were largely demolished, and many of us lost a sense of what 'the future' meant. We became stuck in the present, looking back at the past. For Bryon's clients, this caused a re-emergence of traumatic memories that often led to nightmares combining bad past experiences with the uncertainty and dread of catching coronavirus. The dreams, though, could be used to help some of these people. As Bryon explains, 'Dreams are helping us to transcend a time and space continuum, providing us with structure to metabolize the feelings that are emerging as we live together amidst the ongoing pandemic and political unrest.'[23] In taking their dreams to a psychoanalyst, turning them into a structured narrative and finding links between their past and worry over the future, some clients were better able to make positive plans for their life, Bryon found. By talking about our dreams, we process them, and in turn process a small part of whatever negative emotion or experience fuelled the dream in the first place.

☆ ☆ ☆

There's a particular kind of dream that has attracted a great deal of interest and research over the last few decades. Lucid dreams. Perhaps you've experienced them yourself; a typical dream involves and absorbs us, but in a lucid dream we become suddenly, acutely aware that we're dreaming. The dreamer can then manipulate the dream, living out their wildest fantasies in a euphoric rush. It sounds bonkers if you've never had this happen to you, but I can assure you it is a real phenomenon. I get them quite often, so I can vouch for their existence, but recently, using brain-scanning technology, scientists have been able to prove the re-emergence of consciousness while the mind is still firmly asleep. In the following chapter, we will dive into the strange world of the lucid dream.

Chapter 7

Lucid dreaming

At Aberystwyth University, where I work, there is a peace-ful path and playing field behind the science buildings. One chilly afternoon in late autumn, I was there with some colleagues from an after-work cycling club. We'd just finished a circuit around campus and were chatting as we pushed our bikes towards the car park. It had been a difficult and muddy ride, and we were all soaked to the bone and caked in dirt and grass. The sky was overcast, thick with grey clouds, and the sun would soon be setting.

As I was fiddling with the fastening on my helmet, the leader of our group turned to me.

'Make sure you get cleaned up before you go inside,' he said.

'Will do.'

We walked along the path together. I picked grass off the side of my muddy leg, and wondered if the estates team would be planting a wildflower border like they did last year. After a few minutes of walking, we came out by the Institute of Biology, Earth and Rural Sciences building, the group drifting apart and finishing up conversations as we prepared to go our separate ways.

My feet stopped. The leader of the group continued walking, not noticing my sudden pause. But a creeping feeling had settled in with the damp and cold: something wasn't right with this scene. My head suddenly felt strange – foggy and full of questions. When did I join this club? I haven't ridden a bike since childhood, so whose bike was this? Who were these people, waving and saying 'see you next week'?

The bike wasn't mine, I became certain of that. I wasn't a member of a cycling club. I couldn't name the club's leader, now disappearing up the path. Yet everything else seemed intensely real. The ground felt solid beneath my feet and a cold wind grazed my cheeks. Llandinam Building on my left looked as grey and weird as it always did; I could see someone climbing the steps outside. I stretched out my hand and touched the wall next to me, felt its rough concrete against my fingers. I gripped the worn handlebars of the bike more tightly, as though trying to squeeze out the truth of the matter. I was close. I almost had it.

When it finally came, the realisation was like a static shock. This was a dream.

I was awake, covered in mud, leaning on the handlebars of a bicycle, outside the IBERS building on a gloomy autumn afternoon. But I wasn't there at all; I was in bed nearly a mile down the road, still dreaming. And I could also recall that this was not the first time it had happened to me, either.

Then came the rush of excitement that never lessens with each experience. I was *dreaming*. I could do anything I wanted; the bike could have fold-out wings and I could cycle to the Moon. I could leap into the group-leader's arms and he'd whisk me away to Venice. I could let a T. rex loose on campus. The thrill of limitless freedom woke me up.

This is the phenomenon known as lucid dreaming. You become aware that you're dreaming while the dream is still taking place; sometimes, with practice, you can then assert control over the dream's content. A study conducted in Germany in 2011 found that 51% of participants had experienced this at least once in their lives, making it a rather common parasomnia in the general population.[1] Unlike other parasomnias, though, they tend to be welcomed and sometimes even actively encouraged in our sleeping lives. There are numerous reasons why people want to develop the ability to lucid dream. As we'll explore in this chapter, there is growing evidence of the benefits of being able to control our dreams, including new methods of therapy, fine-tuning motor skills, enhancing creativity, and a sense of spiritual enlightenment. It has been described for centuries, but for people who've never experienced it, it can be difficult to accept that lucid dreaming is real. With the availability of technology to observe brain waves during sleep, however, neuroscientists have been able to prove its existence.

☆ ☆ ☆

Lucid dreaming, particularly its potential for creativity and its sensation of freedom, has been cultivated in Buddhist meditation and Hindu yoga practices since the early medieval period. It is often discussed in terms of spiritual ascension or an otherworldly power, as well as being a physiological phenomenon. Common to both theories, however, is one aspect in particular: the ability to experience lucid dreams can be learned.

In the early 1980s, lucid dreaming as a practised skill or form of mental exercise received a renewal of interest in Western psychology and neuroscience. At the forefront of this wave of research was Stephen LaBerge, an American psychophysiologist who was influenced by a 1975 experiment designed by Keith Hearne and published in the journal of the Society for Psychical Research. Hearne investigated whether regular lucid dreamers could control their rapid eye movement (REM) while dreaming, thus sending a signal to witnesses. As explained in Chapter 4, sleep paralysis ensures we don't usually act out our dreams, but our eyes still follow the patterns of whatever we're looking at in the dream. While undertaking his PhD in the 1980s, LaBerge developed Hearne's experiment; he asked a group of experienced and reliable lucid dreamers to move their eyes in a certain rhythm when they realised they were dreaming. It was a pattern that could not be mistaken for the unpredictable movement of REM. Then, while observing the group asleep, he watched as their eyes made the signal that they were lucid within a dream. Not only did his experiment help to prove the reality of lucid dreams, it also suggested that lucid dreamers are able to control their muscle activity from within the dream.[2]

In 1985, LaBerge wrote a book for a popular readership entitled *Lucid Dreaming: The power of being aware and awake in your dreams*. The same year, he designed a prototype for a device (the 'DreamLight') that aimed to induce lucid dreams electronically. It worked as a mask over the eyes that, during REM sleep, would flash small lights into the eyes of the sleeper. The theory was that the dream would incorporate these lights in some shape or form, and the sleeper would recognise the cues and become lucid. Testing the prototype on a group of fourteen subjects in 1995, LaBerge and co-investigator Lynne Levitan found that eleven of them reported lucid dreams while wearing the mask. The test involved two situations; on some nights the participants wore a switched-off device in bed, and on others they received light cues from the DreamLight during REM sleep. For the nights when the device was set to flash, the participants reported fifteen times more lucid dreams over the study period than nights when the light function was deactivated.[3] But, as LaBerge explains, 'There is little chance of developing a device that will *make* you have lucid dreams – you must bring something of yourself to the effort.' In other words, in order for a device like this to be successful, you have to demonstrate skill in being able to recognise when you're in a dream. Later in the chapter, we'll investigate some of the more modern advances in technology designed to measure and induce lucid dreaming.

☆ ☆ ☆

LaBerge's work may have contributed to scientific proof of humans' ability to lucid dream, but stories about this phenomenon can be found from centuries ago. There's an interesting report, for example, of a lucid dream that dates from 1740. Reprinted in Frank Seafield's *The Literature and Curiosity of Dreams* (1869), it's an extract of a letter written by an 'eminent divine', published in *The Scot's Magazine* in 1763. The unnamed man is writing to Andrew Baxter, author of *An Enquiry into the Nature of the Human Soul* (1730), about some strange experiences he has had in his dreams.[4]

'I am frequently troubled with frightful dreams,' he writes. He goes on to say that because of these nightmares, he has 'gained a kind of habit reflecting how the case stands with me, and whether I be awake or asleep.' By becoming lucid, the man becomes 'indifferent' to the dream. It no longer scares him. He realises that the things he fears in his dreams can't hurt him, and that he can choose whether to watch the scene play out or to end the dream completely and wake up. 'This, you will say, is extraordinary,' he says to Baxter. We don't have Baxter's reply, so can only guess what he made of it.

Also in Seafield's treasure-trove of lucid dreams is an article of 1836 from the *Dublin University Magazine*, which includes an exciting, and really quite funny, discussion of lucid dreaming by the anonymous contributor. It describes in detail the only time the writer experienced a lucid dream:

> 'Here, to all appearance, we are,' we exclaimed; 'the streets are redolent with life around us; the firm earth is reso-nant under our boot – the sun hath a saffron, but clear brightness in Heaven – and yet all this is the merest sham – for we are at this moment at home in our own bedchamber, a thousand miles from hence. What is to withhold us, if we please, from annihilating this proud city by the breath of our nostrils?'

This description reminds me of the countless times I've looked around in a dream, completely bewildered by the idea that this tactile imitation of reality is happening inside my head. It's also interesting that among the author's initial reactions is a destruc-tive impulse. The omnipotent quality of lucid dreams is enticing. Yet there's also something child-like about the experience. I have fond memories as a child of building intricate houses out of

Lego, which I would then gleefully smash with a plastic dinosaur. Lucid dreaming can feel a little bit like that, sometimes. The contributor signs off, to my great amusement, with an offer to Robert Macnish to republish his anecdote in the next edition of *The Philosophy of Sleep* 'for a trifling gratuity'. I hope he'd have settled for appearing in this book, instead.

The term 'lucid dream' seems to have first appeared in 1913. Frederick van Eeden, in his essay 'A Study of Dreams', written for the Society for Psychical Research, sought to explore the 'poetical function' of dreaming.[5] He splits his dreams into distinct types, such as 'original dreams', 'pathological dreams' and 'wrong waking up', and lists their causes, frequency and effects. Among this list is the 'lucid dream', which van Eeden describes as 'highly pleasant' and 'very beneficial, sometimes premonitory'.

Further in the essay, van Eeden explains in detail what he means by this specific type of dreaming. If dreams involve a kind of dislocation from our normal waking selves, then van Eeden argues that lucid dreaming reintegrates these separate parts of our life. He describes the feeling of having a double memory, of the waking mind inhabiting the 'dream-body'. In my lucid dreams, one of the things I can never fully comprehend is this sensation of being in two places at once. As van Eeden writes, 'When I see the blue sky in a lucid dream, I see it as clearly, as brightly, as consciously as I now see this paper.'

The notion of the 'dream-body' was expanded into the realms of pseudoscience by Sylvan Muldoon, a twentieth-century American esotericist who was keenly interested in ideas of astral projection. His book, *The Projection of the Astral Body* (1929), combines emerging theories of lucid dreaming with the notion that the self could transcend the body in sleep.

Of the dream body, he writes that it 'is nothing more nor less than the astral body in partially conscious condition.'[6] The purpose of lucid dreaming, for Muldoon, is to try to push the dream body out of the physical body.

Prior to LaBerge's crucial work, a woman named Mary Arnold-Forster was conducting her own innovative experiments in lucid dreaming. The culmination of this work was her book, *Studies in Dreams*, published in 1921. Arnold-Forster examines various aspects of dreaming, interrogates Freud's theories of interpretation, and discusses the war imagery still lingering in people's sleep from the First World War. In terms of lucid dreaming, though, she was ahead of her time – it only seems to be in the last few decades, more recently fuelled by Christopher Nolan's film *Inception* (2010), that lucid dreaming has become a part of popular discussion.

Arnold-Forster explores her own lucid dreams in depth, presenting them matter-of-factly and without trying to defend the reality of her experience. This was what she dreamed, and it was real to her. She writes:

> On various occasions long ago, when a dream of grief or terror was becoming intolerably acute, the thought flashed into my sleeping mind, 'This is only a dream; if you wake, it will be over, and all will be well again.' If only we could ensure the realisation of this fact directly bad dreams appeared, they would cease to have any terrors for us, for a way of escape would always be open. Therefore I tried repeating this formula to myself from time to time, during the day and on going to bed, always in the same words – 'Remember this is a dream. You are

to dream no longer' – until, I suppose, the suggestion that I wanted to imprint upon the dream mind became more definite and more powerful than the impression of any dream; so that when a dream of distress begins to trouble me, the oft-repeated formula is automatically suggested and I say at once: 'You know this is a dream; you shall dream no longer – you are to wake.' For a time after this secret had been fully learned, this would always awaken me at once; nowadays, the formula having been said, I do not have to wake, though I may do so, but the original fear dream always ceases. It is simply 'switched off', and a continuation of the dream, but without the disturbing element, takes its place and goes forward without a break.[7]

Throughout her exploration into lucid dreams, Arnold-Forster returns to the idea of it being a 'learned secret'. One of the things LaBerge emphasises in his work is the ability to improve the frequency and duration of lucid dreams, so it's interesting that Arnold-Forster presents a precursor to this. While she wasn't the first to identify that lucid dreams could be a practised skill – many cultures and religions, from Mayan to Native American to Chinese antiquity, used lucid dreaming as part of a spiritual rite of passage – she does present an early case of using lucid dreams for more secular, individual reasons. Arnold-Forster demonstrates a clear purpose for lucid dreams: banishing nightmares. A proposal of hers that is particularly resonant is that 'in the early years of childhood most of us could easily be taught simple methods of [dream] control.' The methods she describes are what are now called 'reality checks' – small actions or phrases repeated throughout the day that are designed to make you question reality. If practised enough, the intention is that you'll dream about questioning reality, too, and that will spur you into becoming lucid. We'll return to this idea later in the chapter. For Arnold-Forster, though, her habit is to remind herself periodically that she is dreaming and should wake up, even when she's not asleep. The mantra would then return to her during a nightmare, successfully pulling her out of it. If we all did this, she says, we could stop bad dreams – and the distress that comes with them – before they start. Thinking back to how long it took me to overcome my childhood fear of the dark after my alien nightmare, would I have improved more quickly if education about dreams was more mainstream? If I could have learnt to lucid dream before the bad dreams started, I'd have let the aliens get eaten by a T. rex.

LaBerge's interest was largely in proving the existence of lucid dreams and as a tool for spiritual exploration. Lucid dreaming is now beginning to be explored as a form of therapy, which perhaps Arnold-Forster would have encouraged. Studies are being done on patients suffering with post-traumatic stress disorders, particularly soldiers and veterans, to see how their nightmares might be treated through practising lucid dream induction techniques. Known as 'imagery rehearsal therapy' (IRT), the premise is that patients actively engage with their nightmares during the day while also participating in whichever lucid dream induction technique works best for them – we'll explore these methods later in the chapter. Rather than ignoring the effects of their recurrent traumatic dreams, patients translate them into narratives, try to self-analyse them or identify regular dream signs. Several studies ask participants to reimagine how these dreams end; instead of culminating in something horrible, patients rewrite the dream so that an explosive device spews marshmallows or their car flies up into the air the second before it collides with a tree.

In a 2016 study led by Gerlinde C. Harb, researchers tested imagery rehearsal therapy with soldiers suffering PTSD from serving in US operations in the Middle East between 2001 and 2014.[8] These soldiers reported recurrent nightmares that would continue to shake them in the daytime. After encouraging them to develop a habit of rewriting their nightmares, the team found something interesting. While the number of nightmares suffered by the participants didn't decrease, the soldiers found that they were less distressed by them because they could influence the direction of the dream and rescript the narrative much more often than before the trial. In other words, IRT restored a sense of 'mastery' to an aspect of their lives that they previously thought they could not control. Harb's research has led to subsequent IRT trials. In 2019, UK researchers led by Justin Havens reported on their programme of nightmare-rescripting for 92 military veterans. One group of participants received training on imagery rehearsal therapy, while another group was given advice on 'sleep hygiene' (regular bedtimes, limiting screen time before bed). Prior to the sessions, the participants' nightmares were measured on various scales, such as the 'Nightmare Assessment Scale'. One month after the programme of IRT or sleep hygiene training, their nightmares were reassessed. Havens' team, corroborating Harb's, found a clinically significant reduction in the severity of nightmares for those who had received imagery rehearsal therapy. For the sleep hygiene group, the change was minimal. Moreover, 76% of the IRT group reported in their feedback that they had ideas for how to continue to apply rescripting techniques to their nightmares.[9]

These trials are exciting in the way researchers use creativity – particularly creative writing – in conjunction with dreaming to promote well-being. Throughout the book, we've looked at the relationship between literature and sleep, but in most cases it's in terms of using writing to try to pin down the indescribable aspects of dreams and hallucinations. Indeed, as we saw in the last chapter, there has been discussion about fiction's harmful effects on our dreams. Here, however, writing is used to shape a person's dreaming life for the better; by learning to control the narratives of dreams, it can improve their health.

☆ ☆ ☆

Five years after the release of *Lucid Dreaming*, LaBerge published *Exploring the World of Lucid Dreaming* in collaboration with Howard Rheingold, an American critic with a particular interest in digital methods of communication. This is written as a guide-book, not merely describing what it feels like to lucid dream, but setting out step-by-step instructions to help the reader develop and practise techniques to learn how to do it. LaBerge promotes lucid dreams as the key to 'finding your deepest identity' and to enhance the experience of life. The modern phenomenon of lucid dreaming shares the glamorisation set out by LaBerge. There seems to be a heavy cultural importance applied to productivity at the moment; magazines and online influencers tell us how to work better and study harder, how to set up side-hustles and see every free moment as a chance for self-improvement. Some aspects of lucid dreaming's popularity seem to tie in to this need; if only we could carry on being productive and improving ourselves when we're asleep. A 2013 article in *Men's Fitness* magazine, for instance, bears the title: 'In your dreams: pick up eight more hours of productivity – or something else – through lucid dreaming.' The article calls lucid dreams a 'secret testing ground for honing your skills' and offers three steps to induce this parasomnia.[10] It's all quite misleading – we might sleep for eight hours, but we're certainly not dreaming for the entirety of the night – but the article offers something tantalising to its readers: the chance to rest *and* continue to work on 'that quarterly presentation.'

It's no surprise, then, that this promise of unlocking sleep's potential to help us achieve that lofty goal of super-productivity has a huge online following. One of the most notable examples of this is the Lucid Dreaming page on the multi-forum website Reddit (/r/LucidDreaming). Created in 2009, as of September 2021 it has amassed over 400,000 members, or 'oneironauts' – one of Stephen LaBerge's favourite terms. Indeed, much of the foundations for discussion in this sub-Reddit are taken from the work of LaBerge, who is revered as a sort of leader. It works a little like a continuous extension of *Exploring the World of Lucid Dreaming*, offering advice, anecdotes, problems, and exercises. Members of the community share their successes and experiences, as well as tips for improving the frequency and duration of their lucid dreams. The discussions are always interesting, especially for the fact that many contributors report that they have never experienced a lucid dream before. Lucid dreaming becomes a goal, a white whale, for these particular members; when they post exasperated messages about the months or even years that have passed by without any success in achieving lucidity, other members of the community rally round with comments about persevering. When, at long last, they experience a lucid dream for the first time, they receive dozens of congratulatory messages. Dreaming is such a subjective and personal experience, so it's incredible that lucid dreaming seems to have developed its own public space.

Induction techniques are a key focus of the lucid dreaming community. To delve into the sub-Reddit is to face a plethora of acronyms and codewords, some of which have been taken from LaBerge's work, but others have developed within the sub-Reddit itself. The users of the forum almost have their own language when discussing lucid dreams. But some of the induction techniques do have clinical applications, and there are journal articles about lucid dreaming in which teams of researchers have used a preferred induction technique in their investigation.

There's a particular question that pops up often in online discussions: how did you *learn* to lucid dream? There are several ways to do this, but they share the same characteristic: you have to spend time in your waking hours focusing on what's going to happen when you fall asleep.

'Wake Up, Back to Bed' (WBTB) seems to be one of the most popular induction techniques. This process involves setting an alarm far earlier than you would normally wake up – say 3am if you normally get up at 7am – and spending time awake, somewhere between half an hour and an hour. Promoters of the induction technique specify that it must be a solid amount of time, so not a quick trip to the kitchen for a snack. You're supposed to get out of bed and do something menial, like cleaning, while contemplating lucid dreams and telling yourself that you will become lucid when you fall asleep again. Then, after the time has passed, you go back to bed. The dreams experienced for the rest of the night are then said to be intensely vivid and far more likely to lead to lucidity.

Another popular method is the FILD technique. This acronym stands for Finger Induced Lucid Dream. The theory is that as you drift back to sleep, you lay your hand flat on the mattress. You have to move your index and middle fingers ever so gently, as though you're pressing laptop keys but lightly enough not to push them down. If that makes sense. You'll fall asleep while still concentrating on the repetitive movement of your fingers, and then you'll find you're dreaming without realising it at all.

One of the most common tips on /r/LucidDreaming is to encourage aspiring oneironauts to do 'reality checks' throughout the day. As we saw above, the theory is that if you question reality enough times during the day, you'll remember to do it in your dream – and in your dream, it will be warped in some way and you'll become lucid. This was popularised through the 'totem' object in *Inception*, which we'll return to later; the characters each carried with them a personal token they knew well – its weight, its size, its unique marks – and they would be able to tell they were dreaming if the object felt strange somehow. For Leonardo DiCaprio's character, Cobb, it was a small spinning top that never lost its momentum in dreams. If he spun it and it slowed down and fell over, he knew he was awake.

I don't do reality checks during the day, unless I've come across something bizarre (those 'pinch me, I'm dreaming' moments), but I find them useful to confirm my suspicions when I think I might be dreaming. Sometimes my dreams are so realistic and vivid that I genuinely can't tell if I'm awake or not. I've tried a couple of different methods over the years, with varying success, but the reality check that works best for me is this: in the dream, I pinch my nose, clamp my lips shut and take a deep breath in. Then something weird happens – I feel myself breathing as normal, yet my nose is tightly squished between my finger and thumb. I shouldn't be able to breathe at all. The physiological wrongness of the sensation jolts me, and makes me incredibly lucid and aware of what's around me. And I know, with absolute certainty, that I'm dreaming.

I woke up, for example, to a dream that took place in the bedroom where I had fallen asleep. It was morning, the flock of sparrows that live in the garden hedge were bickering, and I was calm and relaxed as I got out of bed. Then, out of nowhere, I had the idea that I was dreaming. Impulse took over; I wanted to fly up into the welcoming, clear sky, so I opened the window wide and climbed up onto the wooden sill.

But then I stopped. I looked down. Was I absolutely certain this was a dream? There were the birds, hopping around on the grass. I could see the sheep in the field beyond. Nothing was out of place except the feeling I had that it was a dream. If I was wrong, I'd break my leg, or worse. I pinched my nose, and felt my lungs expand with a big gulp of air. I breathed out. It was definitely a dream. I launched myself out of the window and was lifted up like a feather in a warm breeze.

It seems as though lucid dreaming can be learned through paying more attention to the separation between dreams and reality. In addition to periodically questioning reality during waking hours, taking time to write down and reflect on dreams in the daytime can also help people to recall them in more detail. The more vivid dreams become as a result of this practice, the more dream motifs are recognised, thus making it easier for a person to recognise that they're dreaming. As I mentioned in an earlier chapter, this works a little too well for me. I have bursts when I write in a dream diary, but after a few days they balloon into long, labyrinthine sagas that are too weird even for me. But if you're someone who can never quite pin down what you dreamt about, it's worth trying. Even if you just start with a feeling or colour, it may soon build up into something much more vivid – and then you might find yourself becoming lucid, too.

☆ ☆ ☆

In 1956, American philosopher Norman Malcolm disputed the experience of lucid dreaming. 'Of course,' he wrote, 'a person can *dream* that he is sound asleep and can *dream* that he *knows* that he is sound asleep. It can be said of a person who dreamt either of these things that "he knew in his dream" that he was sound asleep. What my argument proves is that knowing-in-your-dream that you are sound asleep is not knowing that you are sound asleep.'[11] I bet he was great fun at parties.

When we dream, we exhibit rapid eye movement (REM). During this stage, our brain waves, as depicted in MRI scans, are of the most basic form of consciousness that only focuses on the present. That's why we never consider how we get to the dream situation; we're plunged into the middle of something and accept our role until we wake up. But in a lucid dream, brain waves belonging to waking consciousness are also exhibited. We can think about things beyond what we're immediately perceiving in a dream, reflecting on the past and the future, and realising that what we're experiencing isn't real.

In other words, it's now difficult to conclude that someone was simply dreaming about being lucid. The brain patterns provide evidence: the lucid dreamer regains waking consciousness while still within the dream. It's important to note, though, that there is an overlap. The basic brain waves of REM sleep – that narrow focus on the immediate moment – are still present despite the sudden spike of waking consciousness. I can certainly feel it; there's a sense of urgency in a lucid dream, as though I have no time to choose what I want to explore because the pull of normal dreaming passivity is getting stronger every moment. I act on impulse, and usually seek the immediate thrill of flying if I don't feel able to assert much control over the dream.

In 2014, a team led by Ursula Voss – one of the leading neuroscientists exploring lucid dreaming – published a paper in *Nature Neuroscience* investigating the re-emergence of waking consciousness in dreams.[12] Specifically, they looked at whether the brain waves exhibited in a normal dream could be influenced by external stimulation. While measuring a sleeper's brain activity as they experienced a lucid dream, Voss's team found an increase of 40 Hz in lower gamma brain waves – an aspect of the brain's function associated with intelligence levels, learning, and memory. By stimulating a normal dreamer with a similar frequency, they found that brain waves began to exhibit the patterns of a lucid dream. They then woke up the participant and asked them to describe their dream, and they reported a distinct increase in the level of conscious awareness.

This research, in development with the practice of lucid dreaming to treat nightmares, could soon provide an innovative therapeutic technique. But the uses of lucid dreaming don't end there; scientists are working to explore its potential for improving creativity, to help athletes practise their sport even in sleep, or to ease social anxiety and the fear of public speaking.

Our acceptance of the delusion of dreams can seem like something of an unbreakable barrier; our waking and dreaming selves seem entirely separate. In lucid dreams, that wall is removed. It's like coming to the surface of a deep swimming pool; the muffled light and sound and sluggish movement suddenly breaks away into a crisp awareness of the world around you. It's extraordinary. The dream opens up, and anything is possible.

Anything that makes some sort of narrative sense, that is. I don't know if this is the same for other lucid dreamers, but I can't just make things appear or completely change the scene like a movie transition. I have to bring it in naturally. But this excites me; one of my favourite things about lucid dreaming is that it can be a little bit like a game or a writing exercise. Perhaps it's because I teach Creative Writing, but I'm intrigued by the way I have to come up with a path for the dream to take.

Take for example a dream I had in which the setting was a cemetery. It was nothing scary – I remember it being a very bright and vivid dream with blue sky and green grass – but cemeteries aren't terribly fun places. For some reason, I realised I was dreaming. Sometimes this does happen spontaneously, although not as frequently as when I'm having a distressing dream. There was no one around, and the cemetery was quite large; in the time it took me to walk to the gate beyond, I'd have probably woken up. I couldn't just transport myself somewhere a bit more exciting. But I could create a path to a new place.

'I have a pen in my back pocket,' I said. I reached behind me, and found a chunky black marker pen exactly where I said it would be.

I took the pen and moved to a grimy-white wall of a large tomb. I drew a door on the rock, opened the door, and fell face-first onto the balcony of an impressive library.

Sometimes, though, my dreaming brain resists the things I'm trying to create. One of my tricks to bring a person into the dream is to stick my hand behind my back and announce their name. I'll feel a strong, vivid touch of a hand grasping mine, and then I'll guide them around in front of me. It's as creepy as it sounds, and it doesn't always work the way I want it to.

I might, for example, put my hand behind my back and declare that Bette Davis has arrived to give me spicy wisdom in between cigarettes. I'll feel a cold hand around mine, and look to see that there's no one there.

Lucid dreams, then, can be slippery things that combine our wildest imaginations with the reality of the laws of physics. If our control over them isn't absolutely perfect, then it can lead to some rather odd sensations and situations.

☆ ☆ ☆

Over the past decade or so, coinciding with and reciprocating the online forums we saw earlier, lucid dreaming has gained an enormous following in popular culture. Science fiction novels and films, in particular, explore the ways in which lucid dreaming is assisted by technology with inevitable nefarious consequences.

Satoshi Kon's 2006 animated cult classic, *Paprika* (based on a novel of the same name by Yasutaka Tsutsui) centres its plot around a prototype device, the 'DC Mini', that clips onto the sleeper's head like a Bluetooth headset. It allows the sleeper's dreams to be live-streamed to a computer, and, when someone sleeps side-by-side with a user of a DC Mini, they can enter and share each other's dream.

The function of the DC Mini is rather akin to the development of image rehearsal therapy. The protagonist, Dr Atsuko Chiba, enters the dreams of others under the guise of her alter ego, Paprika, to try to demystify the content and soothe the dreamer – she asks what various images represent, and talks the dreams through with the dreamer as they happen. The film opens with Paprika witnessing the dream of a police detective, Toshimi Konakawa. No matter where the dream starts, it always ends the same: Konakawa fruitlessly chases a faceless man down a red-carpeted corridor until the floor wobbles and warps beneath him, dissolving him out of the dream. Konakawa's dreams feature recurrent symbols of movies and film-directing; Paprika teases out these tropes, asking questions and trying to encourage Konakawa to remember his past and who the faceless man is. By controlling the dream and analysing it as it happens, Konakawa recalls his old friend – they were both cinema buffs – who made a short film about two men chasing each other. The friend passed away before the film could be finished, and Konakawa's recurring dream is finally untangled as lingering, unprocessed grief.

One of the most intriguing aspects of *Paprika* is that the characters do seem to become a different version of themselves in the dream world. Their unconscious selves come out into the light, for better or worse. In the world of dreams, Atsuko transforms from a rather cold and reserved personality into Paprika, a sprightly, creative and energetic young woman. Atsuko's traits are still very much there, though, in Paprika's sharp mind and quick decision-making; later in the film, we see a little more of Paprika's warmth come out in Atsuko, too.[13]

But while we see the wonders of lucid dreaming tantalisingly presented in *Paprika*, from Konakawa's successful dream-therapy to the sheer joy of Paprika hopping from a rocket to a flying cloud to a tropical scene on a billboard, the main narrative hints at something darker. Because the DC Mini is a prototype, it is flawed, and allows *too much* access into people's dreams. As such, when a couple of prototypes go missing, dreams and reality begin to blur in a very dangerous removal of the boundary between sleep and wakefulness.

Four years later, in 2010, Christopher Nolan released his blockbuster hit, *Inception*. There are plenty of parallels to *Paprika*, but *Inception* poses the idea of lucid dream technology being used by the military to train and rehearse battle scen-arios, rather than for therapeutic purposes. In the case of the plot, however, the technology has been misappropriated by a band of con-artists to perform a psychological heist from within their target's dream. *Inception* isn't quite as gloriously bizarre as *Paprika*, but it still communicates the strange physics of lucid dreams – especially the creative problem-solving required to change the course of the dream. Nothing in *Inception* 'appears' as if by magic; the odd things happen organically, woven into the sequence of events. The film explores layers of dreams; the idea that, while lucid, we can 'fall asleep' again and dream within a dream. The danger, of course, is that the deeper you go the further away you get from waking reality. *Inception*, like *Paprika*, poses not just a dilemma of technology intruding in our dreams, but of the existential crisis we might face when technology helps us to control our dreams too well. If a device guarantees that we can descend into our own fantasy world, would it affect the way we experience our waking lives?

Lucid dreaming is clearly the current centre of attention when it comes to developing our understanding of sleep. What we have to watch out for, as both of these films warn, is allowing technology to damage the separation between reality and dreams.

☆ ☆ ☆

Alongside research into the therapeutic potential of lucid dreams, there have been experiments and studies looking at the creative and performance benefits of the phenomenon. For example, numerous papers have recently been published which look at the ways lucid dreaming might improve the motor skills of athletes. As previously explained, when we dream, our brains still generate the movement signals that correspond with whatever we're doing, although they're inhibited by the state of paralysis that accompanies REM sleep. With this in mind, a lucid dream could provide the space for extra practice with nearly as much neurological benefit as waking practice.

In 2017, a team of researchers at Heidelberg University in Germany published a paper on their pilot study in this field.[14] Led by Melanie Schädlich, the experiment looked at how lucid dreaming might improve the performance of people learning to throw darts. They invited a group of frequent (i.e., more than once a month) lucid dreamers, and asked them to demonstrate their darts skills with their non-dominant hand. A control group of people who had never experienced a lucid dream also carried out the same test. Then, when asleep, the lucid dream group were asked to divert the dream into a situation where they could continue to practise playing darts. Upon waking, their dart-throwing skills were tested again.

The results are fascinating. Some of the lucid dreamers reported being 'distracted' in the dream, throwing pencils rather than darts, for example, or not having enough control over the objects or events, and they showed no improvement in the test the following morning. However, the more experienced lucid dreamers who maintained good control over the situation and managed to spend some time throwing darts in a realistic manner demonstrated an average increase of 18% in their darts score. This experiment was a pilot study, but perhaps we'll see further research done into the measurable benefits of lucid dreaming on motor skills.

A subsequent study from Schädlich and co-author Daniel Erlacher, however, looked at the *perceived* advantages of lucid dreaming for athletes which, when a large part of sport is down to motivation and mindset, might be just as important. In this report, sixteen athletes were interviewed about how they use lucid dreams to improve their performance in a range of activities from juggling to Alpine skiing. Eleven interviewees stated that they used lucid dreaming with the intention of improving their physical performance – to practise their sport within the dream or gear themselves up for a big competition. For these athletes, lucid dreaming was a positive, important and complementary part of their performance. Two participants said they learnt taekwondo and judo moves more quickly than normal because they continued to practise in their lucid dreams. Another participant controlled their dream to make a friend appear and give them a pep talk, delivering a confidence boost before a big martial arts competition.[15] While more work needs to be done to measure the effect of lucid dreams on skilled performance, this article provides a strong sense that it is invaluable for the dreamers' perceived confidence, well-being and accomplishments.

The relationship between video games and lucid dreams is also being explored by researchers. As we've already seen, there are numerous advantages to lucid dreaming, such as fewer or less troubling nightmares, creative inspiration, and enhanced motor skills. The research being done at the moment seems to be trying to pinpoint exactly how lucid dreams occur, and why, and ways in which they might be strengthened, taught, or induced. Video games feature prominently in many of these studies. A team led by Marc Sestir, for example, undertook a study in 2019 to identify whether people who frequently played games were more likely to experience a lucid dream.[16] They surveyed 291 college students, not just looking for correlations between video game playing and lucid dreaming, but also investigating whether a particular genre of video game led to more frequent lucid dreams.

The study found that participants who played at least once a week experienced control and awareness in their dreams more often than those who did not play as regularly, but in a rather particular and interesting manner. What Sestir's team discovered was that the participants who played games more often dreamt *about* the video game; dreaming about the game would lead to ideas of playing and control, and therefore ideas of lucidity. The gamers weren't necessarily becoming lucid in their dreams in a spontaneous manner; it was only when they dreamt about the game they'd been playing that they associated the experience with being able to choose their own path.

Another discovery they made was that video games involving more immersive physical imagery and gameplay – for example, first-person action games or games requiring physical activity beyond moving fingers on a controller – led to a greater likelihood of dreaming about the game's content than puzzles or two-dimensional platform games. In other words, the more closely the image on the screen resembled a realistic view of the world, the more likely the player would dream about it, and then become lucid in their dream.

☆　☆　☆

From everything we've seen in this chapter, there seems to be one clear, over-arching theme: the sense of exciting potential. There is so much that lucid dreams are being revealed to offer, from enhanced creativity, to a form of therapy, to a way of practising fine motor skills. Sleep researchers are still investigating whether there is any downside to lucid dreams, but so far there is no evidence to suggest this. A report published in 2021 by Tadas Stumbrys of Vilnius University, Lithuania, discussed an experiment to measure possible detrimental effects of lucid dreaming. A group of 489 regular lucid dreamers completed a survey on how the phenomenon impacted their sleep quality, feelings of dissociation, and overall mental well-being. Just 10% of the reports described lucid dreaming as a negative experience, and largely the results showed *better* well-being and a higher degree of feeling refreshed in the morning after a lucid dream.[17]

This is exciting, and demonstrates the potential that lucid dreaming has to encourage creativity, sharpen our motor skills, and improve our well-being. Reading these stories and experiments about the benefits of this parasomnia is inspiring, and it makes me want to put more effort into practising the art of dream control. And that's what the current research seems to be doing: finding ways of perfecting the induction and stability of lucid dreams, setting pre-determined scenarios, and developing technology that both teaches and measures this under-used part of our dreaming experience.

There is still so much work to be done on lucid dreams, however, and so many projects are just getting started. Elsewhere, though, parasomnias are being examined to find new causes, effects and treatments. With the COVID-19 pandemic playing havoc with people's dreams and sleep, too, new studies are being undertaken to understand our nocturnal lives in ever greater depth.

Conclusion

O ver the course of this book, we've looked to past ideas of parasomnias and examined our present understanding; sometimes we've seen outstanding developments in treatment and representation, and at other times we've found ourselves still in the dark. We've witnessed how sharing stories about troubled sleep has led to misunderstandings and stigmatisation, but also how they can capture moments in history, form the basis of thrilling fictional scenarios, and how they can be used in therapeutic practice. But how will our relationship with sleep change in the future? In particular, as we continue to learn more and more about the brain's function in sleep, it's interesting to speculate how technology might influence the way we experience and describe our parasomnias.

The video game industry, for example, is becoming more closely aligned with sleep science. As we saw in the previous chapter, video games can now be so incredibly immersive, especially with the proliferation of virtual-reality headsets, that the experience of playing them can feel like a lucid dream. And in turn, lucid dreams feel like playing a virtual-reality video game. This growing relationship between games and dreams may be crucial in understanding sleep in the future. For example, we could use video games to help improve treatment for certain sleep disorders and conditions that affect sleep such as PTSD and depression. This is something that Patrick McNamara and his team have been investigating since 2018.[1] Previous studies have shown that gamers with a penchant for violent, war-themed video games seem to have far fewer nightmares than the general population. As we've seen, imagery rehearsal therapy is one of the major forms of treatment for troubled sleep still being developed. However, there is still an aspect of forcing the patient to confront their trauma or their fear. IRT has some parallels with playing video games: there's the aspect of control, but also of repeating a stage or level if you lose, changing your tactics and getting better until you overcome the obstacle. With this in mind, could there be a way to use the general idea of IRT with the relaxed escapism of video games?

With this question in mind, McNamara's team created a game called ReScript to be run on a virtual-reality headset. They exposed participants to generic threatening imagery and asked them to change the frightening aspects. The screen inside the headset would display a scary image – things like skulls, dark woods, a person with a knife – and the participant, using controls activated by their own hand movements, could alter the image to make it less threatening. Participants could daub paint on the images to cover over anything they didn't like, turn it into something amusing, resize it or remove it altogether. The researchers give an example of one participant who, faced with a shark, edited it to have what looked like a smiley face. The important thing was that the participant had control over how they received and responded to the image.

While the pilot study was small, with nineteen participants, McNamara's team found evidence among them of a significant reduction in general waking anxiety caused by nightmares. The nightmares of the participants were less severe and, perhaps more importantly, less frequent. By the end of the programme's eight sessions, for example, nightmare distress was an average of 44% lower than at the start of the study. In addition, the researchers found that the language used to describe participants' dreams changed, too. As the programme progressed, the dream reports had fewer words related to anxiety, and more verbs – suggesting that a greater sense of agency was felt by the participants. And this result occurred without making participants directly face the traumatic or unpleasant events that gave them nightmares in the first place. The ReScript team are continuing to develop their programme for follow-up studies in the near future.

Technology might thus be a way to benefit our dreams and calm them, allowing us to have a little more agency over what we see and do when we're asleep. But is there a risk of technology intervening too far into our sleeping lives? In 2013, a team of neuroscientists in Japan reported their results of an experiment to 'decode' dreams.[2] Led by T. Horikawa, the team focused on hypnagogic imagery – the flashes of scenes and pictures seen in an early stage of sleep – and continuously woke their subjects up when they were experiencing this phenomenon. They gathered fMRI data during this stage of sleep, isolating particular patterns in accordance with the images described by the subject on waking. For example, if the subject said they first saw a car, the team isolated a pattern on the data and labelled it as 'car'. By repeating this process, the team could build up a bank, called WordNet, of images and their corresponding brain patterns. They could then predict what the study's participants were dreaming about based on the patterns they had previously recorded. The mean decoding accuracy, they say, was 60%. The article states: 'Together, our findings provide evidence that specific contents of visual experience during sleep are represented by, and can be read out from, visual cortical activity patterns shared with stimulus representation.' There are limitations to this discovery: the subjects' patterns were unique to them, and thus the data for 'car' was different for every dreamer, and the WordNet relied on subjects accurately reporting their own dream narratives. It's not quite the stuff of dream infiltration we saw in *Inception* and *Paprika*, but it does propose that part of the future of sleep research could involve quantifying subjective experiences of parasomnias. As we've seen throughout this book, there are a lot of benefits – social, cultural, and in relation to well-being – in talking about our sleep stories. How will our attitude to sleep change when the content of our dreams, nightmares and hallucinations can be read from a graph, without embellishment or redaction? Especially for people who don't usually remember their dreams, would it feel like an intrusion to have them described by a computer or a team of researchers?

This question is reminiscent of one of Ursula Le Guin's science fiction novels, *The Lathe of Heaven* (1971), in which the protagonist, a man named Orr, can change reality in accordance with his dreams.[3] He has no control over this mysterious power, but finds himself exploited by the man he trusts to help him: his psychiatrist, Dr William Haber. Orr visits Haber for help with his disturbing dreams, and Haber soon uncovers the extent of Orr's ability. The psychiatrist begins Orr's 'treatment':

hypnotising the patient and giving him suggestions to move his dream in a certain direction – one that benefits Haber's career and success. However, Le Guin emphasises the untameable nature of dreams in the book, and Orr's power soon causes chaos. He inadvertently wipes out whole populations, and invites a race of aliens from the star Aldebaran to take over the world. It's an odd little novel, but shows a creeping anxiety of what might happen when psychiatry steps too far into our personal dream-lives.

Sleep isn't just about the number of hours, the time it takes to nod off, or whether you snore or not. Sleep is about stories. It's about monsters and ghosts, desires, aggression, trauma and anxiety, health, creativity, and the state of our inner lives. While I was working on this book, I found that people were encouraged to share with me their own tales of sleep paralysis or hallucinations. At the end of the conversation, we both felt less weird and alone in what we've experienced. The importance of exchanging sleep stories is a key part of the research being undertaken by the DreamsID (Dreams – Interpreted and Drawn) project between Swansea University and Goldsmiths, University of London. Led by Mark Blagrove and Julia Lockheart, DreamsID investigates how talking about dreams and representing them in art can encourage empathy. Their 2021 article describes a study involving 26 pairs of participants; in each pair, the 'dream sharer' would tell their dream to the 'dream discusser'. They found that the dream discussers, on average, demonstrated a significant increase in empathy after listening to their partner's dream. One of the key things, though, was that the dream discussers were told to imagine and describe their feelings if *they* had experienced the dream, and then the dream discusser read the sharer's dream back to them.[4] Rather than passively listen to someone else's dream out of politeness, then, the DreamsID team encourage us to participate more deeply in the exchange of sleep stories. If we do this, then we might realise that our strange sleep isn't so strange after all.

For the immediate future, this is how we should change the way we describe our sleep: for the small-talk question of 'Did you sleep well?' to have more answers than simply the number of hours spent unconscious. Conversations about sleep should embrace the weirdness, too. Of course insomnia is important to talk about, but so are sleep paralysis, lucid dreams and hallucinations. Our little upheavals or our major traumas can all come back through the trapdoor of sleep, so to ignore this part of ourselves can mean that we never really face what our dreams are telling us. They can show us our emotional responses and how things have hurt us more clearly than we can sometimes admit to ourselves during the day. These parasomnias might result from trauma, but they can help us overcome it, too. Our sleep demons tell us so much about ourselves, and perhaps it's time to listen.

Acknowledgements

My heartfelt thanks go to my family: the Vernons, Garthwaites, Doyles and Reids. Thank you for your endless kindness and patience. To Mum, for tucking me back in bed when I'd gone walkabout. To the baby-gate, for making sure I never launched myself down the stairs. To Alfred: thanks for keeping watch through the night.

Thank you to Donald Winchester and everyone at Watson, Little literary agency for welcoming me and being so enthusiastic about the book, and to my editor, Kiera, and everyone at Icon Books. I hope I haven't given you too many nightmares.

My colleagues and students at Aberystwyth University are a wonderful bunch, and I'm grateful for the advice, wisdom and encouragement you all gave me while writing this book. I'd especially like to thank Jacqueline, for always being cool and helping me to see that the world isn't so terrifying after all. I'm also grateful for the support of pals across the globe, past and present: Lucy, Alex, Vicky, Millie, Robyn, Cassie, Kath and Dave, Tiffany, Jeremy and Gill.

This book is also dedicated to anyone who's ever told me about their weird dreams. Keep them coming.

References

ABC 11 Eyewitness News, 'Joseph Mitchell found not guilty in "sleepwalking" murder trial', 12 March 2015, https://abc11.com/joseph-mitchell-blake-attempted-murder-jury/553824/

Adams, Allen J., 'Remarkable Case of Somnambulism', *Chicago Medical Journal*, Vol. 26, 1869, 650–55

Adler, Shelley, *Sleep Paralysis: Night-mares, Nocebos, and the Mind-Body Connection* (New Brunswick, NJ: Rutgers University Press, 2011)

American Society for Psychical Research, 'Notes of a Sitting with Planchette', *Journal of the American Society for Psychical Research*, Vol. 2 (11), 1908, 627–40

Arnold-Forster, Mary, *Studies in Dreams* (London: George Allen & Unwin Ltd, 1921)

Bassetti, Claudio, Silvano Vella, Filippo Donati, Peter Wielepp, Bruno Weder, 'SPECT during sleepwalking', *The Lancet*, 356, 2000, 484–5

Beaumont, John, *An Historical, Physiological and Theological Treatise of Spirits, Apparitions, Witchcrafts and Other Magical Practices* (London: D. Browne, 1705)

Belden, L.W., *An Account of Jane C. Rider, the Springfield Somnambulist* (Springfield, CT: G. and C. Merriam, 1834)

Bjorvatn, Bjørn, Janne Grønli, Ståle Pallesen, 'Prevalence of different parasomnias in the general population', *Sleep Medicine*, 11, 2010, 1031–34

Blagrove, Mark, Sioned Hale, Julia Lockheart, Michelle Carr, Alex Jones, Katja Valli, 'Testing the Empathy Theory of Dreaming: The

Relationships Between Dream Sharing and Trait and State Empathy', *Frontiers in Psychology*, Vol. 10, 2019, 1–13

Bond, John, *An Essay on the Incubus, or Night-mare* (London: D. Wilson and T. Durham, 1753)

Brierre de Boismont, Alexandre, *On Hallucinations: A History and Explanation, or, Apparitions, Visions, Dreams, Ecstasy, Magnetism and Somnambulism*, trans. by Robert T. Hulme (London: Henry Renshaw, 1859)

Brontë, Charlotte, *Jane Eyre* (London: Wordsworth Editions, 1999)

Bulwer Lytton, Edward, 'The Haunted and the Haunters: or, The House and the Brain', *The Penguin Book of Ghost Stories* (London: Penguin, 2010), 39–66

Christie, Agatha, *An Autobiography* (London: HarperCollins, 2010 [1977])

Crowe, Catherine, *The Night Side of Nature, or, Ghosts and Ghost Seers* (London: George Routledge and Sons, 1866)

Dalí, Salvador, 'Dream Caused by the Flight of a Bee Around a Pomegranate a Second Before Awakening', 1944, Thyssen-Bornemisza Museum

Davies, Owen, 'The Nightmare Experience, Sleep Paralysis and Witchcraft Accusations', *Folklore*, 114(2), 2003, 181–203

Dickens, Charles, *A Christmas Carol* (London: Macmillan & Co. Ltd, 1922)

van Eeden, Frederick, 'A Study of Dreams', *Proceedings of the Society for Psychical Research*, Vol. 26, (Glasgow: Robert Maclehose & Company Ltd, 1913), 431–61

Ferriar, John, *An Essay Towards a Theory of Apparitions* (London: Cadell and Davies, 1813)

Freud, Sigmund, *The Interpretation of Dreams* (Ware: Wordsworth Editions Ltd, 1997)

Freud, Sigmund, *Beyond the Pleasure Principle*, Second Edition (London: The Hogarth Press, 1942)

Gray, Robert, *The Theory of Dreams*, Vol. 1 (London: F.C. and J. Rivington, 1808)

Le Guin, Ursula, *The Lathe of Heaven* (London: Gollancz, 2001)

Gurney, Edmund, F.W.H. Myers, Frank Podmore, *Phantasms of the Living* Vol. 1 (London: Trübner and Co., 1886)

Hammond, William A., MD, *Sleep and its Derangements* (Philadelphia: J.B. Lippincott & Co., 1869)

Harb, Gerlinde C., Janeese A. Brownlow and Richard J. Ross, 'Posttraumatic Nightmares and Imagery Rehearsal: The Possible Role of Lucid Dreaming', *Dreaming*, 26:3, (2016), 238–49

Hardy, Thomas, *Tess of the D'Urbervilles* (London: Penguin Classics, 2003)

Harris, William V., *Dreams and Experience in Classical Antiquity* (Cambridge, MA: Harvard University Press, 2009)

Havens, Justin, Jamie Hacker Hughes, Fiona McMaster, and Roger Kingerlee, 'Planned Dream Interventions: A Pragmatic Randomized Control Trial to Evaluate a Psychological Treatment for Traumatic Nightmares in UK Military Veterans', *Military Behavioral Health*, Vol. 7(4), 2019, 401–13

Hearn, Lafcadio, 'Yuki-Onna', *Oriental Ghost Stories* (Ware: Wordsworth Editions Ltd, 2007), 79–84

Hearn, Lafcadio, 'Nightmare-Touch', *Shadowings* (London: Kegan Paul, Trench, Trübner & Co. Ltd, 1905), 235–48

Hitchcock, Alfred (dir.), *Spellbound* (Selznick International Pictures, 1945)

Horikawa, T., M. Tamaki, Y. Miyawaki, Y. Kamitani, 'Neural Decoding of Visual Imagery During Sleep', *Science*, 340:6132, 2013, 639–42

Hunter, Elizabeth, 'The Noctambuli: tales of sleepwalkers and secrets of the body in seventeenth-century England', *The Seventeenth Century*, 37(1), 2022, 99–124

Jackson, Shirley, 'The Tooth', *The Lottery and Other Stories* (London: Penguin Classics, 2009), 265–86

James, M.R., 'Oh, Whistle, and I'll Come to You, My Lad', *The Penguin Book of Ghost Stories* (London: Penguin, 2010), 261–80

The Journal of the Anthropological Institute of Great Britain and Ireland, Vol. 18 (London: Trübner & Co., 1888), 135–7

Kon, Satoshi (dir.), *Paprika* (Sony Pictures Entertainment Japan, 2006)

LaBerge, Stephen and Howard Rheingold, *Exploring the World of Lucid Dreaming* (New York: Ballantine Books, 1990)

Langston Parker, S.W., *On the Effects of Certain Mental and Bodily States Upon the Imagination* (Birmingham: Josiah Allen, 1876)

Lask, Bryan, 'Novel and non-toxic treatment for night terrors', *BMJ: British Medical Journal*, Vol. 297 (6648), 1988, 592

Lewis-Hanna, Lourence L., Michael D. Hunter, Tom F.D. Farrow, Iain D. Wilkinson, Peter W.R. Woodruff, 'Enhanced cortical effects of auditory stimulation and auditory attention in healthy individuals prone to auditory hallucinations during partial wakefulness', *NeuroImage*, 57, 2011, 1154–61

LondonDeejay, Tripadvisor, July 2009, https://www.tripadvisor.co.uk/Hotel_Review-g528825-d573931-Reviews-The_Wellington_Hotel-Boscastle_Cornwall_England.html (accessed 19 May 2021)

MacCurdy, John T., *War Neuroses* (Utica, NY: State Hospitals Press, 1918)

MacKay, Cassidy and Teresa L. DeCicco, 'Pandemic Dreaming: The Effect of COVID-19 on Dream Imagery, a Pilot Study', *Dreaming*, 13(3), 2020, 222–34

MacLehose, William F., 'Captivating thoughts: nocturnal pollution, imagination and the sleeping mind in the twelfth and thirteenth centuries', *Journal of Medieval History*, 2020, 46:1, 98–131

Malcolm, Norman, 'Dreaming and Skepticism' (originally published in *Philosophical Review*, 1956), *Philosophical Essays on Dreaming*, ed. by Charles E.M. Dunlop (Ithaca; London: Cornell University Press, 1977), 103–26

de Manacéïne, Marie, *Sleep: Its Physiology, Pathology, Hygiene, and Psychology* (London: Walter Scott, Ltd, 1897)

Mass Observation Online, *Bad Dreams and Nightmares*, http://www.massobservation.amdigital.co.uk/Documents/Details/FileReport-A20 (accessed 9 July 2021)

Mass Observation Online, *DREAMS*, http://www.massobservation.amdigital.co.uk/Documents/Details/FileReport-3096 (accessed 22 September 2021)

McNally, Richard J. and Susan A. Clancy, 'Sleep Paralysis, Sexual Abuse, and Space Alien Abduction', *Transcultural Psychiatry*, 2005, 42(1), 113–22

McNamara, Patrick, Kendra Holt Moore, Yiannis Papelis, Saikou Diallo, Welsey J. Wildman, 'Virtual Reality-Enabled Treatment of Nightmares', *Dreaming*, 28(3), 2018, 205–24

Mendez, Mario F., 'Pavor nocturnus from a brainstem glioma', *Journal of Neurology, Neurosurgery and Psychiatry*, 1992, 860

Morris, Steven, 'Devoted husband who strangled wife in his sleep walks free from court', *The Guardian*, 20 November 2009, https://www.the guardian.com/uk/2009/nov/20/brian-thomas-dream-strangler-tragedy

Muldoon, Sylvan J., *The Projection of the Astral Body* (New York: Samuel Wiser, 1973 [1929])

Muris, Peter, Harald Merckelbach, Thomas H. Ollendick, Neville J. King, Nicole Bogie, 'Children's nighttime fears: parent-child ratings of frequency, content, origins, coping behaviors and severity', *Behavior Research and Therapy*, 2001, 39, 13–28

Murzyn, Eva, 'Do we only dream in colour? A comparison of reported dream colour in younger and older adults with different experience of black and white media', *Consciousness and Cognition*, 17, 2008, 1228–37

Myers, F.W.H., 'The Subliminal Consciousness', *Proceedings of the Society for Psychical Research*, Vol. 7 (London: Kegan Paul, Trench, Trübner & Co. Ltd, 1892), 298–355

Myers, F.W.H., *Human Personality and its Survival of Bodily Death*, Vol 1. (London: Longman, Green, and Co., 1920 [1903])

Ohayon, Maurice M., 'Prevalence of hallucinations and their pathological associations in the general public', *Psychiatry Research*, 97, 2000, 153–64

Old Bailey Proceedings Online (www.oldbaileyonline.org, version 8.0, 8 September 2021), June 1853, trial of SARAH MINCHIN (t18530613-725)

Old Bailey Proceedings Online (www.oldbaileyonline.org, version 8.0, 8 September 2021), September 1876, trial of ELIZABETH CARR (t18760918-413)

Oluwole, O.S.A., 'Lifetime prevalence and incidence of parasomnias in a population of young adult Nigerians', *Journal of Neurology*, 257, 2010, 1141–47

Peters, Ellis, *The Devil's Novice* (London: Sphere, 2011 [1983])

Proceedings of the Society for Psychical Research, Vol. 10 (London: Kegan Paul, Trench, Trübner and Co. Ltd, 1894)

Sacks, Oliver, *Hallucinations* (London: Pan Macmillan, 2013)

Schädlich, Melanie, Daniel Erlacher and Michael Schredl, 'Improvement of darts performance following lucid dream practice depends on the number of distractions while rehearsing within the dream – a sleep laboratory pilot study', *Journal of Sports Sciences*, 2017, 35(23), 2365–72

Schädlich, Melanie and Daniel Erlacher, 'Practicing sports in lucid dreams – characteristics, effects, implications', *Current Issues in Sport Science*, 3, 2018, 1–14

Schenck, Carlos H., Scott R. Bundlie, Milton G. Ettinger, Mark W. Mahowald, 'Chronic Behavioral Disorders of Human REM Sleep: A New Category of Parasomnia', *Sleep*, 9(2), 1986, 293–308

Schmitt, Jean-Claude, 'The Liminality and Centrality of Dreams in the Medieval West', *Dream Cultures: Explorations in the Comparative History of Dreaming*, ed. by David Shulman and Guy G. Stroumsa (New York; Oxford: Oxford University Press), 274–87

Schredl, Michael and Daniel Erlacher, 'Frequency of Lucid Dreaming in a Representative German Sample', *Perceptual and Motor Skills*, 2011, 112(1), 104–08

Scot, Reginald, *The Discoverie of Witchcraft* (London: Elliot Stock, 1886 [1584])

Sestir, Marc, Ming Tai, Jennifer Peszka, 'Relationships Between Video Game Play Factors and Frequency of Lucid and Control Dreaming Experiences', *Dreaming*, 29(2), 2019, 127–43

Shakespeare, William, *Macbeth*, Act 2 Scene 2, L. 34 (New York: W.W. Norton & Company, Inc., 2008), 2569–2632

Sharpless, Brian A., Jacques P. Barber, 'Lifetime prevalence rates of sleep paralysis: A systematic review', *Sleep Medicine Reviews*, 15, 2011, 311–15

Starkey, Marian L., *The Devil in Massachusetts* (New York: Anchor Books, 1969 [1949])

Stevenson, Robert Louis, 'A Chapter on Dreams', *Across the Plains* (London: Chatto & Windus, 1892)

Stevenson, Robert Louis, 'The Strange Case of Dr Jekyll and Mr Hyde', *The Strange Case of Dr Jekyll and Mr Hyde and Other Tales of Terror* (London: Penguin, 2002), 2–70

Stumbrys, Tadas, 'Dispelling the Shadows of the Lucid Night: An Exploration of Potential Adverse Effects of Lucid Dreaming', *Psychology of Consciousness: Theory, Research, and Practice*, 2021, 1–12

The Illustrated Police News, 'A Pretty Somnambulist', 21:534, (Boston, MA: Illustrated Police News Publishing Company, 1877)

Tiraboschi, Pietro, S. Jann, G. Didator, L. Nobili, P. Proserpio, 'Absence of rapid eye movement sleep with hypnopompic visual hallucinations: A possible harbinger of dementia with Lewy bodies?', *Sleep Medicine*, 14, 2013, 377–79

Tuccillo, Dylan, Jared Zeizel and Thomas Peisel, 'In your dreams: pick up eight more hours of productivity – or something else – through lucid dreaming', *Men's Fitness*, 29(10), 2013

Virginia Library, 'Testimony of Richard Coman v. Bridget Bishop', SWP No. 13-13, http://salem.lib.virginia.edu/n13.html#n13.13 (accessed 19 May 2021)

Voss, Ursula, Romain Holzmann, Allan Hobson, Walter Paulus, Judith Koppehele-Gossel, Ansgar Klimke and Michael A. Nitsche, 'Induction of self awareness in dreams through frontal low current stimulation of gamma activity', *Nature Neuroscience*, 17:6 (2014), 810–14

Waite, Felicity, Elissa Myers, Allison G. Harvey, Colin A. Espie, Helen Startup, Bryony Sheaves and Daniel Freeman, 'Treating Sleep Problems in Patients with Schizophrenia', *Behavioural and Cognitive Psychotherapy*, 44, 2016, 273–87

Waters, Flavie, Jan Dirk Blom, Thien Thanh Dang-Vu, Allan J. Cheyne, Ben Alderson-Day, Peter Woodruff, and Daniel Collerton, 'What Is the Link Between Hallucinations, Dreams, and Hypnagogic-Hypnopompic Experiences?', *Schizophrenia Bulletin*, 42(5), 2016, 1098–1109

Notes

Chapter 1: Introduction

1. Bjørn Bjorvatn, Janne Grønli, Ståle Pallesen, 'Prevalence of different parasomnias in the general population', *Sleep Medicine*, 11, 2010, 1031–34.

2. O.S.A. Oluwole, 'Lifetime prevalence and incidence of parasomnias in a population of young adult Nigerians', *Journal of Neurology*, 257, 2010, 1141–47.

3. Jean-Claude Schmitt, 'The Liminality and Centrality of Dreams in the Medieval West', *Dream Cultures: Explorations in the Comparative History of Dreaming*, ed. David Shulman and Guy G. Stroumsa, (New York; Oxford: Oxford University Press), 274–87, p. 278.

4. William V. Harris, *Dreams and Experience in Classical Antiquity* (Cambridge, MA: Harvard University Press, 2009).

5. Reginald Scot, *The Discoverie of Witchcraft* (London: Elliot Stock, 1886 [1584]), p. 68.

6. Bram Stoker, *Dracula* (London: Penguin Classics, 2003 [1897]), p. 275.

7. Edward Bulwer Lytton, 'The Haunted and the Haunters: or, The House and the Brain', *The Penguin Book of Ghost Stories* (London: Penguin, 2010), 39–66, p. 52.

8. M.R. James, 'Oh, Whistle, and I'll Come to You, My Lad', *The Penguin Book of Ghost Stories* (London: Penguin, 2010), 261–80, p. 279.

Chapter 2: Not guilty on grounds of unconsciousness

1. J. Adams Allen, 'Remarkable Case of Somnambulism', *Chicago Medical Journal*, Vol. 26, 1869, 650–55.

2. Old Bailey Proceedings Online (www.oldbaileyonline.org, version 8.0, 8 September 2021), June 1853, trial of SARAH MINCHIN (t18530613-725).

3. Old Bailey Proceedings Online (www.oldbaileyonline.org, version 8.0, 8 September 2021), September 1876, trial of ELIZABETH CARR (t18760918-413).

4. Steven Morris, 'Devoted husband who strangled wife in his sleep walks free from court', *The Guardian*, 20 November 2009, https://www.theguardian.com/uk/2009/nov/20/brian-thomas-dream-strangler-tragedy

5. *ABC 11 Eyewitness News*, 'Joseph Mitchell found not guilty in "sleepwalking" murder trial', 12 March 2015, https://abc11.com/joseph-mitchell-blake-attempted-murder-jury/553824/

6. L.W. Belden, *An Account of Jane C. Rider, the Springfield Somnambulist* (Springfield, MA: G. and C. Merriam, 1834).

7. Wilkie Collins, 'Mr Policeman and the Cook', *Little Novels* (London: Chatto and Windus, 1887), p. 267.

8. Thomas Hardy, *Tess of the D'Urbervilles* (London: Penguin Classics, 2003), p. 246.

9. Carlos H. Schenck, Scott R. Bundlie, Milton G. Ettinger, Mark W. Mahowald, 'Chronic Behavioral Disorders of Human REM Sleep: A New Category of Parasomnia', *Sleep*, 9(2), 1986, 293–308, p. 293.

10. Claudio Bassetti, Silvano Vella, Filippo Donati, Peter Wielepp, Bruno Weder, 'SPECT during sleepwalking', *The Lancet*, 356, 2000, 484–5.

11. 'A Pretty Somnambulist', *The Illustrated Police News*, 21:534 (Boston, MA: Illustrated Police News Publishing Company, 1877), p. 6.

12. William Shakespeare, *Macbeth*, Act 2, Scene 2, L. 34 (New York: W.W. Norton & Company, Inc., 2008), 2569–2632, p. 2593.

13. Elizabeth Hunter, 'The *Noctambuli*: tales of sleepwalkers and secrets of the body in seventeenth-century England', *The Seventeenth Century*, 37(1), 2022, 99–124, p. 102.

14. Shirley Jackson, 'The Tooth', *The Lottery and Other Stories* (London: Penguin Classics, 2009), pp. 265–86.

15. Shirley Jackson, 'How I Write', *Let Me Tell You* (London: Penguin, 2016), 389–93, pp. 392–3.

Chapter 3: Bedroom ghosts

1. Oliver Sacks, *Hallucinations* (London: Pan Macmillan, 2013), p. 210.
2. Pietro Tiraboschi, S. Jann, G. Didato, L. Nobili, P. Proserpio, 'Absence of rapid eye movement sleep with hypnopompic visual hallucinations: A possible harbinger of dementia with Lewy bodies?', *Sleep Medicine*, 14, 2013, 377–9.
3. Flavie Waters, Jan Dirk Blom, Thien Thanh Dang-Vu, Allan J. Cheyne, Ben Alderson-Day, Peter Woodruff, and Daniel Collerton, 'What Is the Link Between Hallucinations, Dreams, and Hypnagogic-Hypnopompic Experiences?', *Schizophrenia Bulletin*, 42(5), 2016, 1098–1109.
4. Felicity Waite, Elissa Myers, Allison G. Harvey, Colin A. Espie, Helen Startup, Bryony Sheaves and Daniel Freeman, 'Treating Sleep Problems in Patients with Schizophrenia', *Behavioural and Cognitive Psychotherapy*, 44, 2016, 273–87.
5. F.W.H. Myers, 'The Subliminal Consciousness', *Proceedings of the Society for Psychical Research*, Vol. 7 (London: Kegan Paul, Trench, Trübner & Co. Ltd., 1892), 298–355, p. 304.
6. F.W.H. Myers, *Human Personality and its Survival of Bodily Death*, Vol. 1 (London: Longman, Green, and Co., 1920 [1903]), p. 125.
7. Alexandre Brierre de Boismont, *On Hallucinations: A History and Explanation, or, Apparitions, Visions, Dreams, Ecstasy, Magnetism and Somnambulism*, trans. by Robert T. Hulme (London: Henry Renshaw, 1859), p. 450.
8. John Ferriar, *An Essay Towards a Theory of Apparitions* (London: Cadell and Davies, 1813), p. 14.
9. Catherine Crowe, *The Night Side of Nature, or, Ghosts and Ghost Seers* (London: George Routledge and Sons, 1866 [1853]), p. 194.
10. John Beaumont, *An Historical, Physiological and Theological Treatise of Spirits, Apparitions, Witchcrafts, and Other Magical Practices* (London: D. Browne, 1705), p. 197.
11. Lourence L. Lewis-Hanna, Michael D. Hunter, Tom F.D. Farrow, Iain D. Wilkinson, Peter W.R. Woodruff, 'Enhanced cortical effects of auditory stimulation and auditory attention in healthy

individuals prone to auditory hallucinations during partial wakefulness', *NeuroImage*, 57, 2011, 1154–61.

12. Edmund Gurney, Frederic W.H. Myers, Frank Podmore, *Phantasms of the Living* (London: Trübner and Co., 1886), p. 347.

13. *Proceedings of the Society for Psychical Research*, Vol. 10 (London: Kegan Paul, Trench, Trübner and Co. Ltd, 1894), p. 33.

14. John Ruskin, 'The Relation of Art to the Science of Light', *The Eagle's Nest*, 2nd Edition (Orpington: George Allen, 1891), 114–37, p. 123.

15. Maurice M. Ohayon, 'Prevalence of hallucinations and their pathological associations in the general public', *Psychiatry Research*, 97, 2000, 153–64, p. 153.

Chapter 4: Hag-ridden

1. Shelley Adler, *Sleep Paralysis: Night-mares, Nocebos, and the Mind-Body Connection* (New Brunswick, NJ: Rutgers University Press, 2011), p. 2.

2. Owen Davies, 'The Nightmare Experience, Sleep Paralysis and Witchcraft Accusations', *Folklore*, 114(2), 2003, 181–203, p. 184.

3. Marian L. Starkey, *The Devil in Massachusetts* (New York: Anchor Books, 1969 [1949]), p. 54.

4. Virginia Library, 'Testimony of Richard Coman v. Bridget Bishop', SWP No. 13-13, http://salem.lib.virginia.edu/n13.html#n13.13 (accessed 19 May 2021).

5. Reginald Scot, *The Discoverie of Witchcraft* (London: Elliot Stock, 1886 [1584]), p. 68.

6. *The Journal of the Anthropological Institute of Great Britain and Ireland*, Vol. 18 (London: Trübner & Co., 1888), 135–7, p. 136.

7. Charles Dickens, *A Christmas Carol* (London: Macmillan & Co. Ltd., 1922), pp. 18–19.

8. William A. Hammond, MD, *Sleep and its Derangements* (Philadelphia: J.B. Lippincott & Co., 1869), p. 186.

9. John Bond, *An Essay on the Incubus, or Night-mare* (London: D. Wilson and T. Durham, 1753), preface.

10. S.W. Langston Parker, *On the Effects of Certain Mental and Bodily States Upon the Imagination* (Birmingham: Josiah Allen, 1876), pp. 38–9.

11. Edmund Gurney, F.W.H. Myers, Frank Podmore, *Phantasms of the Living*, Vol. 1 (London: Trübner and Co., 1886), p. 454.

12. Lafcadio Hearn, 'Yuki-Onna', *Oriental Ghost Stories* (Ware: Wordsworth Editions Ltd, 2007), 79–84, pp. 82–3.

13. Lafcadio Hearn, 'Nightmare-Touch', *Shadowings* (London: Kegan Paul, Trench, Trübner & Co. Ltd, 1905), 235–48, p. 239.

14. LondonDeejay, TripAdvisor, July 2009, https://www.tripadvisor.co.uk/Hotel_Review-g528825-d573931-Reviews-The_Wellington_Hotel-Boscastle_Cornwall_England.html (accessed 19 May 2021).

15. Richard J. McNally and Susan A. Clancy, 'Sleep Paralysis, Sexual Abuse, and Space Alien Abduction', *Transcultural Psychiatry*, 2005, 42(1), 113–22, p. 115.

Chapter 5: Night terrors

1. 'Notes of a Sitting with Planchette', *Journal of the American Society for Psychical Research*, Vol. 2 (11), 1908, 627–40.

2. Marie de Manacéïne, *Sleep: Its Physiology, Pathology, Hygiene, and Psychology* (London: Walter Scott, Ltd, 1897), pp. 296–7.

3. James Russell, 'Clinical illustrations of the analogy between the processes of health and of disease', *The Medical Times and Gazette*, 1870 (2), 90–92.

4. Ginevra Uguccioni, Jean-Louis Golmard, Alix Noël de Fontréaux, Smaranda Leu-Semenescu, Agnès Brion, Isabelle Arnulf, 'Fight or flight? Dream content during sleepwalking/sleep terrors vs rapid eye movement sleep behavior disorder', *Sleep Medicine*, 2013, 14, 391–8.

5. A.H. Renton, 'On the Poisonous Effects of the Datura Arborea', *Transactions of the Medico-Chirurgical Society of Edinburgh*, 1829, p. 477.

6. Leonard Guthrie, 'On Night Terrors, Symptomatic and Idiopathic, with Associated Disorders in Children', *A System of Medicine*, Vol. 8 (London: Macmillan & Co. Ltd, 1899), 218–37.

7. Charlotte Brontë, *Jane Eyre* (London: Wordsworth Editions, 1999), p. 12.

8. Peter Muris, Harald Merckelbach, Thomas H. Ollendick, Neville J. King, Nicole Bogie, 'Children's nighttime fears: parent-child ratings of frequency, content, origins, coping behaviors and severity', *Behavior Research and Therapy*, 2001, 39, 13–28, p. 18.

9. John T. MacCurdy, *War Neuroses* (Utica, NY: State Hospitals Press, 1918), p. 2.
10. O.F. Aina and O.O. Famuyiwa, '*Ogun Oru*: A Traditional Explanation for Nocturnal Neuropsychiatric Disturbances among the Yoruba of Southwest Nigeria', *Transcultural Psychiatry*, March 2007, 44(1), 44–54, p. 45.
11. Mario F. Mendez, 'Pavor nocturnus from a brainstem glioma', *Journal of Neurology, Neurosurgery and Psychiatry*, 1992, 860.
12. Bryan Lask, 'Novel and non-toxic treatment for night terrors', *BMJ: British Medical Journal*, Vol. 297 (6648), 1988, 592.
13. Agatha Christie, *An Autobiography* (London: HarperCollins, 2010 [1977]), p. 37.
14. Ellis Peters, *The Devil's Novice* (London: Sphere, 2011 [1983]), p. 36.
15. William F. MacLehose, 'Captivating thoughts: nocturnal pollution, imagination and the sleeping mind in the twelfth and thirteenth centuries', *Journal of Medieval History*, 2020, 46:1, 98–131, p. 123.
16. Sean D. Boyden, Martha Pott, Philip T. Starks, 'An evolutionary perspective on night terrors', *Evolution, Medicine, and Public Health*, 2018, 100–05.
17. A.R. Lillywhite, S.J. Wilson and D.J. Nutt, 'Successful Treatment of Night Terrors and Somnambulism with Paroxetine', *British Journal of Psychiatry*, 1994, 164(4), 551–4.

Chapter 6: Narrating dreams

1. Mass Observation Online, *DREAMS*, http://www.massobservation.amdigital.co.uk/Documents/Details/FileReport-3096 (accessed 22 September 2021).
2. Mass Observation Online, *Bad Dreams and Nightmares*, http://www.massobservation.amdigital.co.uk/Documents/Details/FileReport-A20 (accessed 9 July 2021).
3. Robert Gray, *The Theory of Dreams*, Vol. 1 (London: F.C. and J. Rivington, 1808), p. 152.
4. Shane McCorristine, *The Spectral Arctic: A History of Dreams and Ghosts in Polar Exploration* (London: UCL Press, 2018), p. 12.
5. 'Sir John Franklin', *Illustrated London News*, 6 October 1848, p. 227.
6. Wilkie Collins, 'The Frozen Deep', *The Frozen Deep and Other Tales* (London: Chatto & Windus, 1885), 1–136, p. 91.

7. Juvenile Delinquency (Education): Hearings Before the Subcommittee to Investigate Juvenile Delinquency of the Committee on the Judiciary, United States Senate, 1955.

8. 'More Friends for Comics', *Newsweek*, 27 November 1950, p. 50.

9. Robert Louis Stevenson, 'A Chapter on Dreams', *Across the Plains* (London: Chatto & Windus, 1892), p. 248.

10. Robert Louis Stevenson, 'The Strange Case of Dr Jekyll and Mr Hyde', *The Strange Case of Dr Jekyll and Mr Hyde and Other Tales of Terror* (London: Penguin, 2002), 2–70, p. 13.

11. Sigmund Freud, *The Interpretation of Dreams* (Ware: Wordsworth Editions Ltd, 1997), pp. 20–21.

12. *Spellbound*, dir. Alfred Hitchcock (Selznick International Pictures, 1945).

13. Salvador Dalí, 'Dream Caused by the Flight of a Bee Around a Pomegranate a Second Before Awakening', 1944, Thyssen-Bornemisza Museum.

14. Eva Murzyn, 'Do we only dream in colour? A comparison of reported dream colour in younger and older adults with different experience of black and white media', *Consciousness and Cognition*, 17, 2008, 1228–37, pp. 1228–29.

15. Jack Kerouac, *Book of Dreams* (San Francisco: City Lights Books, 1961), pp. 38–9.

16. William S. Burroughs, *My Education: A Book of Dreams* (London: Picador, 1995), p. 40.

17. Sigmund Freud, *Beyond the Pleasure Principle*, Second Edition (London: The Hogarth Press, 1942), p. 44.

18. Antti Revonsuo, 'The Reinterpretation of Dreams: An evolutionary hypothesis of the function of dreaming', *Behavioral and Brain Sciences*, 23, 2000, 877–901, p. 882.

19. Thomas Gregor, 'A Content Analysis of Mehinaku Dreams', *Ethos*, Winter 1981, 9(4), 353–90.

20. Donna Ferguson, '"Last night I was James Bond": the vivid world of lockdown dreams', *The Guardian*, 19 April 2020, https://www.theguardian.com/society/2020/apr/19/last-night-i-was-james-bond-the-vivid-world-of-lockdown-dreams (accessed 28 January 2022); Poppy Noor, 'So you've been having weird dreams during lockdown, too?', *The Guardian*, 23 April 2020, https://www.theguardian.com/lifeandstyle/2020/apr/23/

coronavirus-dreams-what-could-they-mean (accessed 28 January 2022); Eleanor Morgan, 'Our pandemic subconscious: why we seem to be dreaming much more – and often of insects', *The Guardian*, 30 April 2020, https://www.theguardian.com/lifeandstyle/2020/apr/30/our-pandemic-subconscious-why-we-seem-to-be-dreaming-much-more-and-often-of-insects (accessed 28 April 2020).

21. Cassidy MacKay and Teresa L. DeCicco, 'Pandemic Dreaming: The Effect of COVID-19 on Dream Imagery, a Pilot Study', *Dreaming*, 13(3), 2020, 222–34, p. 230.

22. Serena Scarpelli, Valentina Alfonsi, Anastasia Mangiaruga, Alessandro Musetti, Maria Catena Quattropani, Vittorio Lenzo, Maria Francesca Freda, Daniel Lemmo, Elena Vegni, Lidia Borghi, Emanuela Saita, Roberto Cattivelli, Gianluca Castelnuovo, Giuseppe Plazzi, Luigi De Gennaro, Christian Franceschini, 'Pandemic nightmares: Effects on dream activity in the COVID-19 lockdown in Italy', *Journal of Sleep Research*, 2021, 1–10, p. 7.

23. Deborah Bryon, 'Processing trauma and psychoanalysis in "real" time and in dreams: the convergence of past, present and future during COVID-19', *Journal of Analytical Psychology*, 66(3), 2021, 399–410, p. 407.

Chapter 7: Lucid dreaming

1. Michael Schredl and Daniel Erlacher, 'Frequency of Lucid Dreaming in a Representative German Sample', *Perceptual and Motor Skills*, 2011, 112(1), 104–08.

2. Stephen LaBerge and Howard Rheingold, *Exploring the World of Lucid Dreaming* (New York: Ballantine Books, 1990), p. 24.

3. Stephen LaBerge and Lynne Levitan, 'Validity Established of Dream-Light Cues for Eliciting Lucid Dreaming', *Dreaming*, 5(3), 1995, 159–68, p. 167.

4. Frank Seafield, *The Literature and Curiosities of Dreams* (London: Lockwood, 1869), pp. 226–8.

5. Frederick van Eeden, 'A Study of Dreams', *Proceedings of the Society for Psychical Research*, Vol. 26 (Glasgow: Robert MacLehose & Company Ltd, 1913), 431–61, p. 431.

6. Sylvan J. Muldoon, *The Projection of the Astral Body* (New York: Samuel Wiser, 1973 [1929]), p. 163.

7. Mary Arnold-Forster, *Studies in Dreams* (London: George Allen & Unwin Ltd, 1921), p. 56.

8. Gerlinde C. Harb, Janeese A. Brownlow and Richard J. Ross, 'Post-traumatic Nightmares and Imagery Rehearsal: The Possible Role of Lucid Dreaming', *Dreaming*, 26:3, (2016), 238–49.

9. Justin Havens, Jamie Hacker Hughes, Fiona McMaster, and Roger Kingerlee, 'Planned Dream Interventions: A Pragmatic Randomized Control Trial to Evaluate a Psychological Treatment for Traumatic Nightmares in UK Military Veterans', *Military Behavioral Health*, Vol. 7 (4), 2019, 401–13.

10. Dylan Tuccillo, Jared Zeizel and Thomas Peisel, 'In your dreams: pick up eight more hours of productivity – or something else – through lucid dreaming', *Men's Fitness*, 29 (10), 2013.

11. Norman Malcolm, 'Dreaming and Skepticism' (originally published in *Philosophical Review*, 1956), *Philosophical Essays on Dreaming*, ed. by Charles E.M. Dunlop (Ithaca; London: Cornell University Press, 1977), 103–26, pp. 109–10.

12. Ursula Voss, Romain Holzmann, Allan Hobson, Walter Paulus, Judith Koppehele-Gossel, Ansgar Klimke and Michael A. Nitsche, 'Induction of self awareness in dreams through frontal low current stimulation of gamma activity', *Nature Neuroscience*, Vol. 17:6 (2014), 810–14.

13. *Paprika*, dir. Satoshi Kon (Sony Pictures Entertainment Japan, 2006).

14. Melanie Schädlich, Daniel Erlacher and Michael Schredl, 'Improvement of darts performance following lucid dream practice depends on the number of distractions while rehearsing within the dream – a sleep laboratory pilot study', *Journal of Sports Sciences*, 2017, 35(23), 2365–72.

15. Melanie Schädlich and Daniel Erlacher, 'Practicing sports in lucid dreams – characteristics, effects, implications', *Current Issues in Sport Science*, 3, 2018, 1–14.

16. Marc Sestir, Ming Tai, Jennifer Peszka, 'Relationships Between Video Game Play Factors and Frequency of Lucid and Control Dreaming Experiences', *Dreaming*, 29(2), 2019, 127–43.

17. Tadas Stumbrys, 'Dispelling the Shadows of the Lucid Night: An Exploration of Potential Adverse Effects of Lucid Dreaming', *Psychology of Consciousness: Theory, Research, and Practice*, 2021, 1–12, p. 9.

Conclusion
1. Patrick McNamara, Kendra Holt Moore, Yiannis Papelis, Saikou Diallo, Welsey J. Wildman, 'Virtual Reality-Enabled Treatment of Nightmares', *Dreaming*, 28(3), 2018, 205–24.
2. T. Horikawa, M. Tamaki, Y. Miyawaki, Y. Kamitani, 'Neural Decoding of Visual Imagery During Sleep', *Science*, 340: 6132, 2013, 639–42.
3. Ursula Le Guin, *The Lathe of Heaven* (London: Gollancz, 2001).
4. Mark Blagrove, Sioned Hale, Julia Lockheart, Michelle Carr, Alex Jones, Katja Valli, 'Testing the Empathy Theory of Dreaming: The Relationships Between Dream Sharing and Trait and State Empathy', *Frontiers in Psychology*, Vol. 10, 2019, 1–13.

Index

A

Across the Plains (Stevenson) 167
Account of Jane C. Rider, An (Belden)
    38–40
Adams Allen, J. 30–2
Adler, Shelley 91
Aina, O.F. 142–4
Albert the Great, Saint 151
Alice in Wonderland Syndrome 25
American Psychoanalytic Association
    138
antidepressants
    paroxetine 153–4
Arnold-Forster, Mary 206–8
Asclepius 9
astral projection 205–6
Athena 10

B

Bassetti, Claudio 47
Baxter, Andrew 203–4
Beaumont, John 77–8
Belden, L.W. 38–40
belemnites 96

Bellerophon 10
benzodiazepines 147, 151 *see also*
    clonazepam, diazepam
Bergman, Ingrid 172, 173
Beyond the Pleasure Principle (Freud)
    191
Bishop, Bridget 94
Blagrove, Mark 231
Blandy, Frederick 130–1
Bond, John 102–3
Book of Dreams (Kerouac) 180–1
Boyden, Sean D. 152
Brierre de Boismont, Alexandre
    72–3
Brontë, Charlotte 134, 136–7
Brown, Nancy 159
Bryon, Deborah 197–8
Bulwer Lytton, Edward 18
Burroughs, William S. 181–3

C

Cadfael series (Peters) 149–51
Carr, Elizabeth 36
Census of Hallucinations 81–5

253

'Chapter on Dreams, A' (Stevenson)
167–8
Christie, Agatha 148–9
Christmas Carol, A (Dickens) 76,
97
Clancy, Susan A. 120–1
clonazepam 146–7, 148, 154
Collins, Wilkie 41–4, 164
Coman, Richard 94
comic books
    moral panic over 166–7
COVID-19 pandemic 195–8, 225
Cowper, Mr 123, 124
Cowper, Mrs 123
Crowe, Catherine 76–7
Crozier, Francis 162
Cushen, Charles 34–5

D

Dalí, Salvador 173, 181
de Manacéïne, Marie 125
Dean, Mrs G. 157–8
DeCicco, Teresa L. 196
dementia 46–7, 153
    with Lewy bodies 66
Devil's Novice, The (Ellis) 150–1
diazepam 154
Dickens, Charles 76, 97, 164
Discoverie of Witchcraft, The (Scot)
10, 94–5
Doctor Who 11–12
Dracula (Stoker) 14–17, 133
'Dream Caused by the Flight of a Bee'
    (Dalí) 173
dream diaries 180–4
DreamLight 202–3
dreams 8–9, 21–2, 157–98
    animals in 183, 193–4, 196
    in colour 179–80

in COVID-19 pandemic 195–8,
    225
in early human society 192–3
epiphany 8–9
lucid 21–2, 68, 198, 199–225
in Mehinaku tribe 193–4
as portents 160
and psychoanalysis 169–75
'psychic' 161–5
and sleep cycles 160
and sleepwalking 46
DreamsID 231–2
Ducie, Lord 96
Duncan, Andrew 129

E

Eastlake, Elizabeth 76–7
Erebus, HMS 161–2, 164
Erlacher, Daniel 222
*Essay Towards a Theory of Apparitions,
    An* (Ferriar) 74–5
Exploring the World of Lucid Dreaming
    (LaBerge and Rheingold) 210,
    211

F

Famuyiwa, O.O. 142–4
Farthest North (Nansen) 161
Fellini, Federico 180
Ferriar, John 74–5
FILD *see* Finger Induced Lucid
    Dream
Finger Induced Lucid Dream (FILD)
    213
First World War 137–42, 206
Fitzjames, James 162
Franklin, Captain Sir John 161–3
Franklin expedition 161–5

Index

Franklin, Lady Jane 162–3
Freud, Sigmund 21, 161, 169–72,
    191, 206
Frozen Deep, The (Collins) 164–5
Fuseli, Henry 52, 101

G
Good, Sarah 93
Gray, Robert 160
Gregor, Thomas 193–4
Gurney, Edmund 79, 109, 111,
    117
Guthrie, Leonard 132–4

H
Hallucinations (Sacks) 64
hallucinations, hypnogogic 63, 71
hallucinations, hypnopompic 20,
    61–88
    coinage 70, 71
    and dementia 66
    exacerbation by illness 72
    paranormal interpretations 75–7,
        79–85
    and 'micro-arousals' 66
    and schizophrenia 66–7
    sound-based 77–9
Hammond, William 98
Harb, Gerlinde C. 209
Hardy, Thomas 44–5
'Haunted and the Haunters, The'
    (Lytton) 18
Haunting of Hill House, The (Jackson)
    54–5, 56, 57
Havens, Justin 209
Hearn, Patrick Lafcadio 112–16,
    137
Hearne, Keith 202

*Historical, Physiological and Theological
    Treatise of Spirits, An*
    (Beaumont) 77–8
Hitchcock, Alfred 172
Horikawa, T. 229
Hubbard, Elizabeth 93
*Human Personality and its Survival of
    Bodily Death* (Myers) 72
Hunter, Elizabeth 53

I
imagery rehearsal therapy *see* IRT
Inception (Nolan) 22, 206, 213, 220
Incubus, An Essay on the (Bond)
    102–3
Interpretation of Dreams, The (Freud)
    21, 169–72, 180
IRT (imagery rehearsal therapy)
    208–10, 228

J
Jackson, Shirley 54, 55–7
James, M.R. 18
Jane Eyre 134–7

K
Kerouac, Jack 180–1
Kon, Satoshi 22, 218

L
LaBerge, Stephen 202–3, 207, 208,
    210, 211
Langston Parker, S.W. 107
Lask, Bryan 147–8
Lathe of Heaven, The (Le Guin)
    230–1

Le Guin, Ursula 230–1
Levitan, Lynne 203
Lewis-Hanna, Lourence L. 78
Lewy, Friedrich H. 66
Lewy bodies *see* dementia
Lightfoot, Frances 109–12
Literature and Curiosity of Dreams, The (Seafield) 203–4
Lockheart, Julia 231
Lucid Dreaming (LaBerge) 202, 210

M
Macbeth (Shakespeare) 50–2, 53
MacCurdy, John T. 138–42
MacKay, Cassidy 196
Macnish, Robert 46, 165–6, 205
Macrobius 9
Malcolm, Norman 215
'mare-stanes' 96
Mass Observation 157–60
Maury, Alfred 71
McCorristine, Shane 162–4
McNally, Richard J. 120–1
McNamara, Patrick 228–9
Medico-Chirurgical Society of Edinburgh 129
Mehinaku tribe 193–4
melatonin 148
memento mori 83, 108–9
Mendez, Mario 147
'Meredith' 4–8, 21–2, 68–70, 98–101, 184–91
Merrion, Edward 36
Mesmer, Franz Friedrich Anton 40
Millais, John Everett 50
Minchin, Sarah 34–5
Mitchell, Joseph 37
Moonstone, The (Collins) 41, 53, 131

'Mr Policeman and the Cook' (Collins) 41–4
Muldoon, Sylvan 205–6
Muris, Peter 137
My Education (Burroughs) 181–3
Myers, Frederic W.H. 70–2, 79, 109, 111, 117
Mysteries of Udolpho, The (Radcliffe) 97, 165

N
Nansen, Fridtjof 161
Night Side of Nature, The (Crowe) 76–7
'Nightmare, The' (Fuseli) 101
'Nightmare-Touch' (Hearn) 114–16
night terrors 20–1, 64, 122, 123–55
    and epilepsy 126
    and illness/disease 128, 130–1, 133, 153
    and RBD 128–9
    and sleepwalking 128–9
    in war veterans 137–42
    in Yoruba culture 142–4
Nolan, Christopher 22, 206, 220
Northwest Passage *see* Franklin expedition

O
'Oh, Whistle, and I'll Come to You, My Lad' (James) 18
Ohayon, Maurice M. 85
On Hallucinations (Brierre de Boismont) 72–3
'On Night Terrors' (Guthrie) 132–4
On the Effects of Certain Mental and Bodily States Upon the Imagination (Langston Parker) 107–8

'oneironauts' *see* dreams, lucid
Oriental Ghost Stories (Hearn)
    112–14
Osborne, Sarah 93

P

Paprika (Kon) 22, 218–20
parasomnias
    definition 3
    see also dreams, lucid; dreams,
        nightmares; hallucinations,
        hypnopompic; night terrors;
        sleep paralysis; sleepwalking
Pargeter, Edith *see* Peters, Ellis
paroxetine 153–4
Parris, Betty 93
Peters, Ellis 149–51
Phantasms of the Living
    (Gurney et al) 79–81,
    109–12, 117–19
Philosophy of Sleep, The (Macnish) 46,
    165–6, 205
Pliny 9
Podmore, Frank 79, 109, 111, 117
polar exploration 161–5
Polidori, John 166
post-traumatic stress disorder
    (PTSD) 208, 209–10, 228 *see
    also* First World War
'Pretty Somnambulist, A' (*Illustrated
    Police News* report) 49–50,
    52
Prior, Mr and Mrs 49–50
Projection of the Astral Body, The
    (Muldoon) 205–6
psychoanalysis movement 169
PTSD *see* post-traumatic stress
    disorder
Putnam, Ann 93

R

Radcliffe, Ann 97
RBD (REM behaviour disorder)
    46–7, 91, 128–9
Reddit 211–13
Reed, Mrs 111
'Reinterpretation of Dreams, The'
    (Revonsuo) 191–3
REM behaviour disorder *see* RBD
Renton, A.H. 129–32
ReScript 228–9
Revonsuo, Antti 191–3
Rheingold, Howard 210
Rider, Jane C. 38–40, 48
Ruskin, John 83
Russell, James 126–7

S

Sacks, Oliver 64
Salem Witch Trials 10, 93–5
Saunders, Mrs L.H. 80–1
Scarpelli, Serena 197
Schädlich, Melanie 221, 222
Schenck, Carlos 46
schizophrenia 66–7
Scot, Reginald 10, 94–5
Seafield, Frank 203, 204
Second World War 157–60
Sestir, Marc 223
Seymour, Mrs C.R. 80–1
Shadowings (Hearn) 114–16
Shakespeare, William 50
'shell shock' *see* First World War
Sleep (de Manacéïne) 125
Sleep and its Derangements
    (Hammond) 98
sleep paralysis 20, 88, 89–122
    and alien abduction reports
    120–1

sleep paralysis (continued)
    association with witchcraft 92–5
    cause 91–2
    cures 96–8, 103
    in fiction 112–14
Sleep Paralysis (Adler) 91
sleeptalking 58
sleepwalking 19–20, 29–59
    in 19th-century fiction 15–17,
        41–5
    crimes committed while 34–7
    and dreams 46
    and hypnotism 40–1
    noctambulo/'nightwalking' 53
'Sleepwalking Lady Macbeth, The'
    (Fuseli) 52–3
Smith, Frederick 34–5
'Snow Woman' *see* 'Yuki-Onna'
Society for Psychical Research 70–1,
    79, 81, 85, 109, 123–5, 205
somnambulism *see* sleepwalking
'Somnambulist, The' (Millais) 50
Spectral Arctic, The (McCorristine)
    162–4
Speer, Laura 49–50, 52, 53
Spellbound (Hitchcock) 172–5
Starkey, Marian L. 93
Starks, Philip T. 152
Stevenson, Robert Louis 21, 167–9
Stoker, Bram 14, 17
'Strange Case of Dr Jekyll and Mr
    Hyde, The' (Stevenson) 167,
    168–9
Studies in Dreams (Arnold-Forster)
    206–8
'Study of Dreams, A' (van Eeden)
    205
Stumbrys, Tadas 224
'Subliminal Consciousness, The'
    (Myers) 71

T

Terror, HMS 161–2, 164
Tess of the D'Urbervilles (Hardy)
    44–5, 53
Theory of Dreams, The (Gray) 160–1
Thomas, Brian 37
'thought-transference' 80
'thunder stone' 96
Tiraboschi, Pietro 66
Tituba 93
'Tooth, The' (Jackson) 55
TripAdvisor 116–17
Tsutsui, Yasutaka 218

U

Uguccioni, Ginevra 128–9
Unfinished Portrait (Christie) 149

V

van Eeden, Frederick 205
video games 223–4, 227–9
Voss, Ursula 216

W

Waite, Felicity 67, 87–8
'Wake Up, Back to Bed' (WBTB)
    212–13
War Neuroses (MacCurdy) 138–42
Waters, Flavie 66–7, 67–8, 75
WBTB *see* 'Wake Up, Back to Bed'
'Who Killed Zebedee' *see*
    'Mr Policeman and the Cook'
Williams, Abigail 93
WordNet 229–30

Y

Yoruba community 142–4
'Yuki-Onna' (Hearn) 112–14